PHARMACOGNOSY
PRACTICAL NOTEBOOK

for

First Year Diploma in Pharmacy

(According to the new syllabus prescribed by the Pharmacy Council of India, Education Regulation 1991, implemented in the year 1993, for Diploma in Pharmacy Students)

Varun Dutt Sharma M. Pharm.
Principal

S.K. Pandey B. Pharm.
Sr. Lecturer

Janta Polytechnic, Jahangirabad, Bulandshahar, Uttar Pardesh

CBS

CBS Publishers & Distributors Pvt. Ltd.

New Delhi • Bengaluru • Chennai • Kochi • Kolkata • Mumbai
Hyderabad • Nagpur • Patna • Pune • Vijayawada

Pharmacognosy
PRACTICAL NOTEBOOK

ISBN: 81-239-1426-1

First Edition: 2007
Reprint: 2008, 2012, 2014, 2016, 2017, 2018, 2019

Published by **Satish Kumar Jain** and produced by **Varun Jain** for
CBS Publishers & Distributors Pvt. Ltd.,
4819/XI Prahlad Street, 24 Ansari Road, Daryaganj, New Delhi - 110002
delhi@cbspd.com, cbspubs@airtelmail.in • www.cbspd.com
Ph.: 23289259, 23266861, 23266867 • Fax: 011-23243014

Corporate Office: 204 FIE, Industrial Area, Patparganj, Delhi - 110 092
Ph: 49344934 • Fax: 011-49344935
E-mail: publishing@cbspd.com • publicity@cbspd.com

Branches:

- ***Bengaluru:*** 2975, 17th Cross, K.R. Road, Bansankari 2nd Stage, Bengaluru - 70 • Ph: +91-80-26771678/79 • Fax: +91-80-26771680 E-mail: cbsbng@gmail.com, bangalore@cbspd.com
- ***Chennai:*** No. 7, Subbaraya Street, Shenoy Nagar, Chennai - 600030 Ph: +91-44-26681266, 26680620 • Fax: +91-44-42032115 E-mail: chennai@cbspd.com
- ***Kochi:*** Ashana House, 39/1904, A.M. Thomas Road, Valanjambalam, Ernakulum, Kochi • Ph: +91-484-4059061-65 Fax: +91-484-4059065 • E-mail: cochin@cbspd.com
- ***Kolkata:*** 6-B, Ground Floor, Rameshwar Shaw Road, Kolkata - 700014 Ph: +91-33-22891126/7/8 • E-mail: kolkata@cbspd.com
- ***Mumbai:*** 83-C, Dr. E. Moses Road, Worli, Mumbai - 400018 Ph: +91-9833017933, 022-24902340/41 • E-mail: mumbai@cbspd.com

Representatives:

- Hyderabad: 0-9885175004
- Patna: 0-9334159340
- Jharkhand: 0-9811541605
- Nagpur: 0-9021734563
- Pune: 0-9623451994
- Uttarakhand: 0-9716462459

Printed at:
J.S. Offset Printers, Delhi (India)

Certificate

Student's Name ______________________________

Class ____________________ Roll No. ____________

This is to certify that experiments, written in the index, have been performed by the student, are satisfactory.

Grade..................

Name and signature of lab. in-charge

College stamp

Date ....

Preface

The evaluation of crude drug is essential not only at academic lavel but also at large scale in phytochemical, pharmaceutical and perfumery industries. The increasing demand of the crude drug at national and international market may suggest a methodical approach to qualitative and quantitative evaluation of crude drugs in their organized and unorganized forms. The present form of this practical notebook in which crude drugs are classified morphologically according to new syllabus as prescribed by Pharmacy Council of India, Education regulation 1991. This practical notebook contains 70 experiments. The left blank page is provided for making diagram of crude drugs.

We shall be gratefully acknowledged the comments, suggestions and criticisms by respected teachers and students for the improvement of future edition. We express sincere thanks to Mr Satish Kumar Jain and Mr Y.N. Arjuna, M/S CBS Publishers & Distributors for their co-operation, encourgagement and assistance in bringing out the present form of this manual. Finally our greatest gratitude are to our colleagues Mr R.K. Singh and Mr Anil Kumar for their inspiration and motivation. We are also thankful to Sandeep Kumar for sincere co-operation in preparing the typed manuscript of the concern book.

Varun Dutt Sharma • S.K. Pandey

Syllabus

1. Identification of drugs by morphological characters.
2. Physical and chemical tests for evaluation of drugs wherever applicable.
3. Gross anatomical studies (TS) of the following drugs – Senna, Datura, Cinnamon, Cinchona, Coriander, Fennel, Clove, Ginger, Nuxvomica, Ipecacuanha.
4. Idenfitication of fibres and surgical dressings.

Contents

Preface iv

1. List of Apparatus and Instruments 1

2. General Instructions 3

3. Introduction 5

4. Leaf : Identification of Leaf Drugs by Morphological Characters 9

Morphology of leaves
Experiment 1: Senna 15
Experiment 2: Digitalis 17
Experiment 3: Vasaka 19
Experiment 4: Gymnema 21
Experiment 5: Tulsi 23
Experiment 6: Belladonna 25
Experiment 7: Nim 27

5. Bark: Identification of Bark Drugs 29

Morphology of Bark
Experiment 8: Arjuna 33
Experiment 9: Ashok 35
Experiment 10: Cinchona 37
Experiment 11: Cinnamon 39

6. Flower: Identification of Flower Drugs 41

Morphology of Flower
Experiment 12: Clove 43
Experiment 13: Pyrethrum 45

7. Fruit: Identification of Fruit Drugs 47

Morphology of Fruit
Experiment 14: Amla 49
Experiment 15: Coriander 51
Experiment 16: Caraway 53
Experiment 17: Cardamom 55
Experiment 18: Ajowan 57
Experiment 19: Black pepper 59
Experiment 20: Orange peel 61
Experiment 21: Lemon peel 63
Experiment 22: Bahera 65
Experiment 23: Gokhru 67

8. Seed: Identification of Seed Drugs 69

Morphology of Seed
Experiment 24: Isphagula 73
Experiment 25: Nux vomica 75
Experiment 26: Linseed 77
Experiment 27: Nutmeg 79
Experiment 28: Colchicum 81

9. Root and Rhizome: Identification of Root and Rhizome Drugs 83

Morphology of Root and Rhizome
Experiment 29: Aswagandha 85
Experiment 30: Aconite 87
Experiment 31: Ginger 89
Experiment 32: Turmeric 91
Experiment 33: Garlic 93
Experiment 34: Rauwolfia 95
Experiment 35: Rhubarb 97
Experiment 36: Liquorice 99
Experiment 37: Picrorrhiza 101
Experiment 38: Shatavar 103
Experiment 39: Dioscorea 105
Experiment 40: Pippali 107
Experiment 41: Ipecacuanha 109

10. Herb and Whole Plant 111

Morphology of Stem, Leaf, Flower and Fruit
Experiment 42: Shankhapushpi 113
Experiment 43: Punarnava 115
Experiment 44: Ephedra 117
Experiment 45: Cannabis 119
Experiment 46: Vinca 121

11. Wood 123

Morphology of Wood
Experiment 47: Sandal wood 125

12. Gross Anatomical Study *127*

General Description of Plant Tissues (Histology) and Section Cutting

Experiment 48: Senna *131*
Experiment 49: Datura *133*
Experiment 50: Cinchona *135*
Experiment 51: Cinnamon *137*
Experiment 52: Coriander 139
Experiment 53: Fennel *141*
Experiment 54: Clove *143*
Experiment 55: Ginger *145*
Experiment 56: Nux vomica *147*
Experiment 57: Ipecacuanha *149*

13. Identification of Fibers and Surgical Dressing *151*

Experiment 58: Vegetable and regenerated fibres *153*

14. Physical and Chemical Tests for Evaluation of Unorganized Drugs *154*

Physical and Chemical Characters

Experiment 59: Aloes *157*
Experiment 60: Catechu *159*
Experiment 61: Agar *161*
Experiment 62: Acacia *163*
Experiment 63: Tragacanth *165*
Experiment 64: Colophony *167*
Experiment 65: Asafoetida *169*
Experiment 66: Myrrh *171*
Experiment 67: Bees-wax *173*
Experiment 68: Honey *175*
Experiment 69: Castor oil *177*
Experiment 70: Gelatin *179*

INDEX

S. No.	Name of the experiment	Page No.	Remarks

INDEX

S. No.	Name of the experiment	Page No.	Remarks

INDEX

S. No.	Name of the experiment	Page No.	Remarks

INDEX

S. No.	Name of the experiment	Page No.	Remarks

1

List of Apparatus and Instruments

A. List of common equipment use in pharmacognosy laboratory as per ER-91.

	Special equipment and instruments	*Nos. required 60 students*	*For 120 students*
1.	Dissecting microscope	20	20
2.	Charts (different types)	100	100
3.	Models (different types)	50	50
4.	Permanent slides	100	100
5.	Slides and cover slips	Adequate	Adequate

B. List of instruments/equipment for the students which they should bring themselves

1.	Practical manual	1
2.	Slides	2
3.	Cover slips	Adequate
4.	Cello tape	1
5.	Board pins	Adequate
6.	Scissor	1
7.	Blade	1
8.	Pen	1
9.	Pencil HB	1
10.	Rubber	1
11.	Pencil sharpener	1
12.	Scale	1
13.	Dissecting forceps	1
14.	Fractional weight	1 box
15.	Apron	1
16.	Test tubes	Adequate
17.	Butter paper, etc.	Adequate

2

General Instructions

General Instructions

1. Students must read the theory and the technique of the experiment before coming to practical class.
2. Students should wear apron in lab.
3. Bring necessary equipment with them in lab.
4. Every operation should be recorded carefully.
5. Draw diagrams neatly.
6. Each experiment should show the date, experiment no. and object of the experiments.
7. Each experimental record should be duly completed and shown to the teacher for correction and signature.
8. Completed manual is assessed for allotment of marks for "day-to-day work"

With the above in view, the experiments outlines in this manual have been selected and designed to help the students to understand the basic procedures for identification of drugs. The students must learn the idea underlying these experiments, as understanding of these fundamental is necessary for a proper grasp of the subject. The students should do experiments themselves.

3

Introduction

The history of medicine in India can be traced to the remote past. The drugs recorded in Indian medical literature, very few are of mineral and animal origin, while majority of drugs are derived from vegetable sources. The earliest mention of the medicinal use of plants is found in the *Rig Veda* written about 5000 years ago. In the works which follow particularly *Ayurveda*, the properties of various drugs have been given in detail.

Pharmacy: It is the art of preparing, compounding and dispensing drugs, suitable for administration and for the treatment of disease.

Crude drugs

The natural form of drug, not compounded, treated or mixed with any other substances.

Drugs

The chemical agents, which effect living protoplasm and are intended for use in the treatment, prevention or diagnosi of disease.

Pharmacognosy

It is the science, which deals with the source, history, cultivation, collection, as well as physical and chemica characteristics of crude drugs.

Pharmacognosy is not only concerned with naturally occurring substances possess medical action but it is alsc concerned with other subsistence such as pharmaceutical aids which included surgical dressing prepared fron natural fibre, flavouring agents, suspending agents, disintegrating agents, filling and support medium.

Types of drugs action

Stimulation, depression, irritation, substitution or any other selective action.

Sources of crude drugs

(A) Minerals, e.g. talc, kaolin, bentonite, chalk, diatomite and asbestos, etc.
(B) Animals
- (a) Entire animal, e.g. cantharides.
- (b) Part of animal, e.g. thyroid glands.
- (c) Derived from animals (by extraction, etc.), e.g. cod liver oil, gelatin, wax, etc.

(C) Plants
- (a) Entire plants, e.g. Irish moss
- (b) Part of Plants
  - (i) Organized drugs
    - (a) Leaf
    - (b) Flowers or bud

(c) Fruits
(d) Seeds
(e) Bark
(f) Wood
(g) Underground part, e.g. roots or rhizomes

(ii) Unorganized drugs
(a) Gums
(b) Resins
(c) Extracts and juices

(iii) Others: for example fibres and fabrics

Pharmacognostical study includes

(a) Study of origin or source, e.g. biological, geographical, history and name, etc.
(b) To study morphological nature of drug.
(c) To study about cultivation, method of collection, drying, packing and other treatment for preparation to the market.
(d) Description or characteristics: It includes the following:
1. The physical form and dimension of crude drug.
2. The colour, odour and taste of crude drug.
3. The fracture and texture of crude drug.
4. Condition of drug, e.g. fresh or dried.
5. Microscopically and histological characteristics
6. To study about potency and purity of drug.
7. To study about constituents and chemical test for identification of drugs.

I. Morphological classification

(A) According to habitat

(a) Terrestrial: Grow above the ground, e.g.
(b) Aquatic: Grow in water, e.g. lotus.
(c) Epiphytic, e.g. lichens.
(d) Parasitic, e.g. ergot.

(B) According to age

(a) Annuals, e.g. wheat, etc.
(b) Biennials, e.g. carrot, etc.
(c) Perennials, e.g. all trees, etc.

(C) According to structure

(a) Tree
1. Tall tree
2. Medium tree
3. Small tree

(b) Shrubs
(c) Herb
(d) Weak plants
(i) Prostrate
(ii) Twinning plants

(iii) Climbing plants
(iv) Lianas

II. Taxonomical classification: (According to modern concept).

Division, Subdivision, Class, Subclass, Series, Order, Family, Genus, Species, Botanical Name, Local Name

Plant Kingdom

Thallophyta *1 Class*	*Embryophyta* *1*	
Algae	*Bryophyta*	*Tracheophyta*
1. Cyanophyta 2. Euglenophyta 3. Chlorophyta 4. Crysophyta 5. Pyrrophyta 6. Phacophyta 7. Rhodophyta	Musci Hepaticase Anthocrotale Anthocrotae	Prilopsida Lycopsida Sphenopsida Pteroprida
Fungi		Filicineae Gymnospermae Angiospermae
8. Schizomycophyta	sub-order	sub-order
9. Myxomycophyta	Cycatophytae	Dicotyledonae
10. Eumycophyta	Coniterophytae	Monocotyledonae

Description details of plants

1. Habit

(a) Annual or biennial or perennial.
(b) Herb or shrub or tree.

2. Root

Tap root or adventitious root.

3. Stem

Erect or climber or procumbent or decumbent or creeping.

4. Leaf

(a) *Duration:* Caduceus or deciduous or persistent.
(b) *Arrangement on stem:* Spiral or alternate or opposite or whorled.
(c) *Parts of leaf:* Petiolate or sessile.
(d) *Stipules:* Stipulatė, caduceus or persistent or estipulate.
(e) *Shape of lamina:* Acicular, linear, lanceo late, oblong, ovate, cordate, sagittate, hastate, lunate, obviate, obcordate, spathulate, cuneate/tunicate, oval/elliptical, orbicular.
(f) *Apex of lamina:* Acute, acuminate/caudate, obtuse, mucronate, spiny, tendriller, cirrhose, truncate, retuse, emarginate.

(g) *Margin of lamina:* Entire, wavy, serrate, biserrate, retroserrate, dentate, bidentate, crenate, bicrenate, spiny, lobed.
(h) *Base of lamina:* Connate, perfoliate, auriculate-amplixicaul.
(i) *Leaf surface:* Glabrous, hairy, rough, gelatinous, spiny.
(j) *Texture of leaf:* Coriaceous, membranous, fleshy, succulent.
(k) *Venation:* Reticulate venation, parallel venation.
(l) *Type of leaf:* Simple or compound.
 (i) Palmately compound leaf, unifoliate compound leaf or bifoliate compound leaf or trifoliate compound leaf or multifoliate compound leaf.
 (ii) Pinnately compound leaf, unipinnate compound leaf or bipinnate compound leaf or tripinnate compound leaf or decompound leaf.

5. Inflorescence

Racemose or cymose or special or compound.

6. Flower

(a) Pedicellate or sessile.
(b) Complete or incomplete.
(c) Hermaphrodite/bisexual or unisexuale.
(d) Symmetry: Regulate/actinomorphic or monosymmetrical/zygomorphic or asymmetrical/ irregular.

7. Barks

Generally it means all tissues outside the cambium. Normally bark is composed of following tissues.
(i) Epidermis
(ii) Primary cortex
(iii) Endodermis
(iv) Pericycle
(v) Phloem

Bark can be described as follows:

Origin and preparation from trunk, branches or roots, whole or inner bark.

Size and shape

Surface: Lichens, mosses, lenticels, cracks or furrows, colour before and after scraping. Inner surface colour, striations, furrows.

Fracture: Either short or fibrous, granular, etc.

8. Wood

(a) Heart wood or sap wood.
(b) Transverse surface.
(c) Hardness.
(d) Density.
(e) Longitudinal surface.

4

Leaf

Identification of Leaf Drugs by Morphological Characters

Leaves are flat, green and broad part of the shoot which possess neither nodes nor internodes and branches arise in their axils. For morphological study of various crude drugs the following types of characters are studied.

1. Arrangement of leaves (phyllotaxy)

(a) Alternate

Only one leaf arises from each node. Every next leaf arises from the successive node in opposite direction, e.g. peepal.

(b) Opposite

Two leaves are attached at each node opposite to each other, e.g. jasmine.

(c) Whorled

More than two leaves are attached at each node arranged in a whorl, e.g. oleander.

2. Shape

Shape of lamina may be acicular, linear, lanceolate, oblong, subulate, ovate, cordate, sagittate, hastate, reniform, lunate, obovate, obcordate, spathulate, cuneate, elliptical and rotund.

3. Margin

Entire, repend, serrate, biserrate, retroserrate, dentate, bidentate, crenate, bicrenate, spiny and lobed.

4. Apex

Acute, acuminate, obtuse, mucronate, cuspidate, tendrillar, cirrhose, truncate, retuse, emargenate, etc.

5. Petiole

It is leaf stalk which cylindrical or sub-cylindrical structures.

(a) *Petiolate:* A leaf with petiole.
(b) *Sessile:* A leaf without petiole.

6. Surface

(a) *Glabrous:* Smooth surface.
(b) *Pubescent:* Hairy surface.
(c) *Glaucous:* Covered by whitest substances.
(d) *Gland dotted:* Possessing non-sticky glands.
(e) *Spiny:* Covered by spine.

7. Stipule

It is a small outgrowths of the leaf base which protects the young leaves and the axillary buds.
(a) *Stipulate:* Stipule present.
(b) *Exstipulate:* Stipule absent.

8. Venation

Distribution pattern of the veins and veinlets in the lamina of a leaf in called venation.

(a) Reticulate venation

The veinlets are irregularly distributed to form a network, e.g. dicot. plant. It may be unicostate or multicostate. Multicostate venation is of two types—convergent and divergent .

(b) Parallel venation

In this case the veins run parallel to each other and network is not formed, e.g. monocot. plants. It is of two types — unicostate and multicostate.

9. Leaf incision (simple and compound)

(a) Simple leaf

A leaf is said to be simple when its lamina is entire or incised to any depth but not up to the midrib or petiole.

(b) Compound leaf

When incision of the margin is reached to the midrib to form many leaf-like lobes called leaflets which are found on the rachis. The compound leaves are of two types:

(1) Pinnate

Compound leaf in which the rachis is elongated and bears two rows of simple or divided leaflets. It is of the following types.
(i) **Uni-pinnate:** It is of two types.
 (a) *Paripinnate:* The unipinnate leaf with even number of leaflets.
 (b) *Imparipinnate:* The unipinnate leaf with odd number of leaflets, e.g. nim.
(ii) **Bi-pinnate:** The main rachis produces secondary lateral rachis which bears leaflets, e.g. Acacia.
(iii) **Tri-pinnate:** In this case the tertiary rachis bears the leaflets.
(iv) **De-compound:** The incision is of higher order than in tri pinnate, e.g. fennel, coriander, etc.

(2) Palmate compound leaves

Leaflets are attached at the tip of petiole giving an appearance of palm of hand. It is of the following types.
(i) **Uni-foliate:** A single terminal leaf, e.g. lemon.
(ii) **Bi-foliate:** Two leaflet are attached at the terminal end of petiole.
(iii) **Tri-foliate:** This type of leaf has three terminal leaflets, e.g. wood apple.

(iv) Quadri-foliate: The leaf has four leaflets attached to the tip of petiole.
(v) Multi-foliate: The leaf has five or more leaflets arranged as fingers of the palm, e.g. Bombox.

10. Texture

(i) Herbaceous: Delicate.
(ii) Coriaceous: Leathery in touch.
(iii) Succulent: Fleshy and juicy.
(iv) Membranous: Thin flexible and translucent.
(v) Cereous: Waxy.

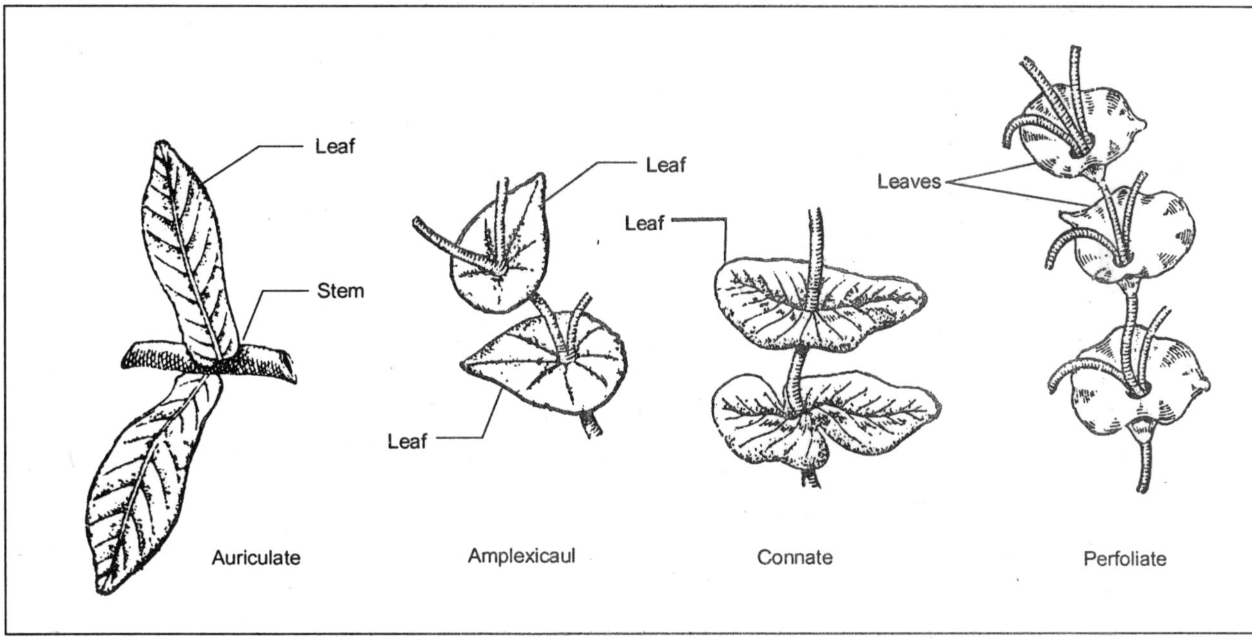

Leaf base

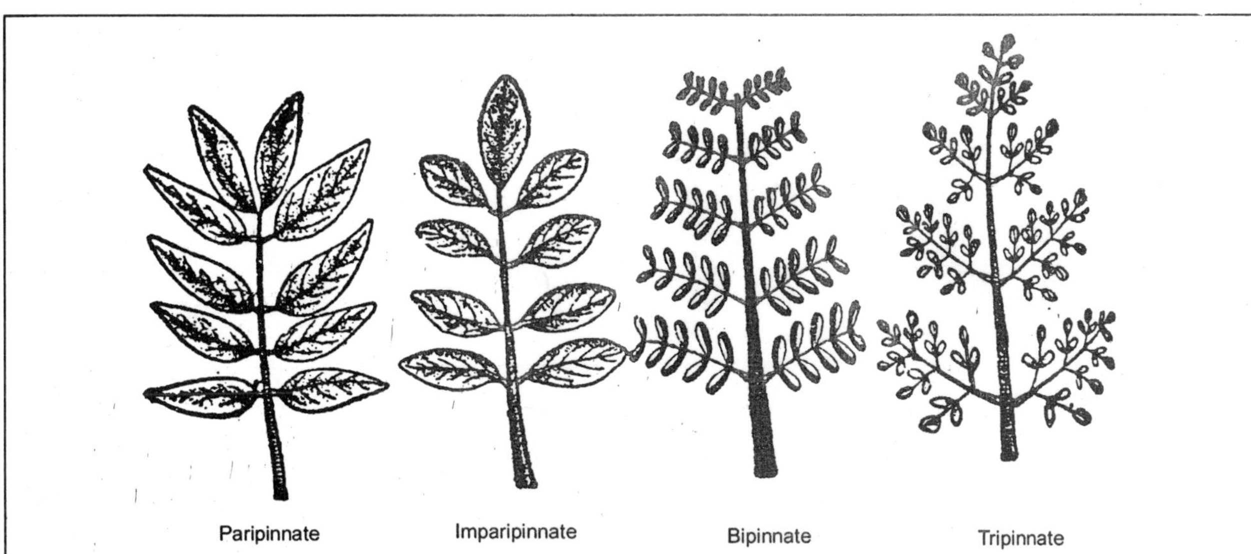

Pinnate compound leaf

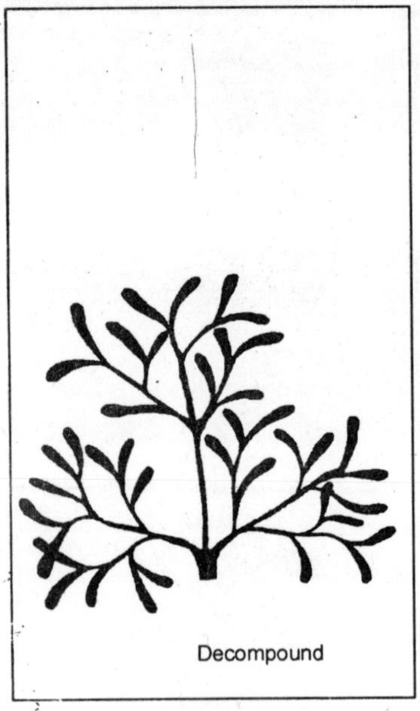

Pinnate compound leaf

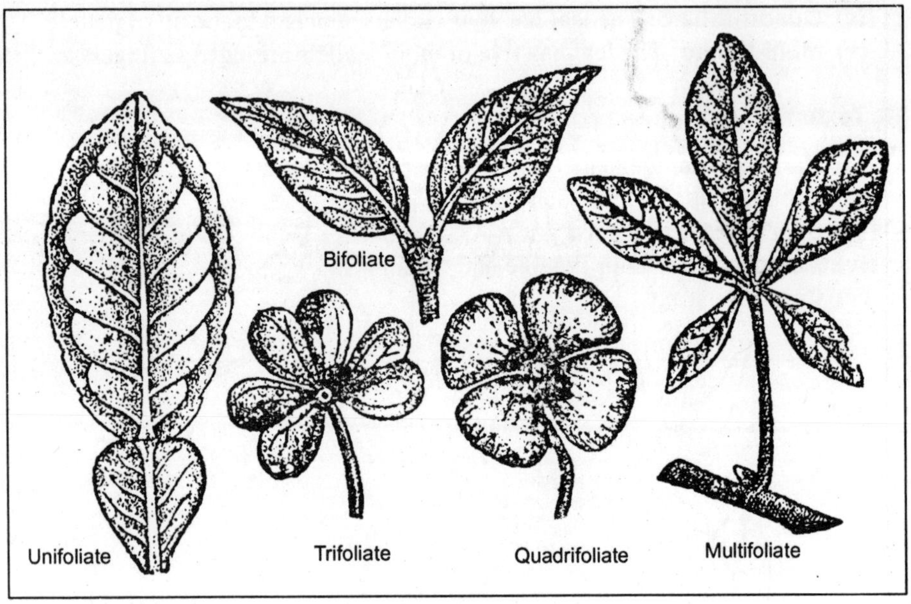

Palmate compound leaf

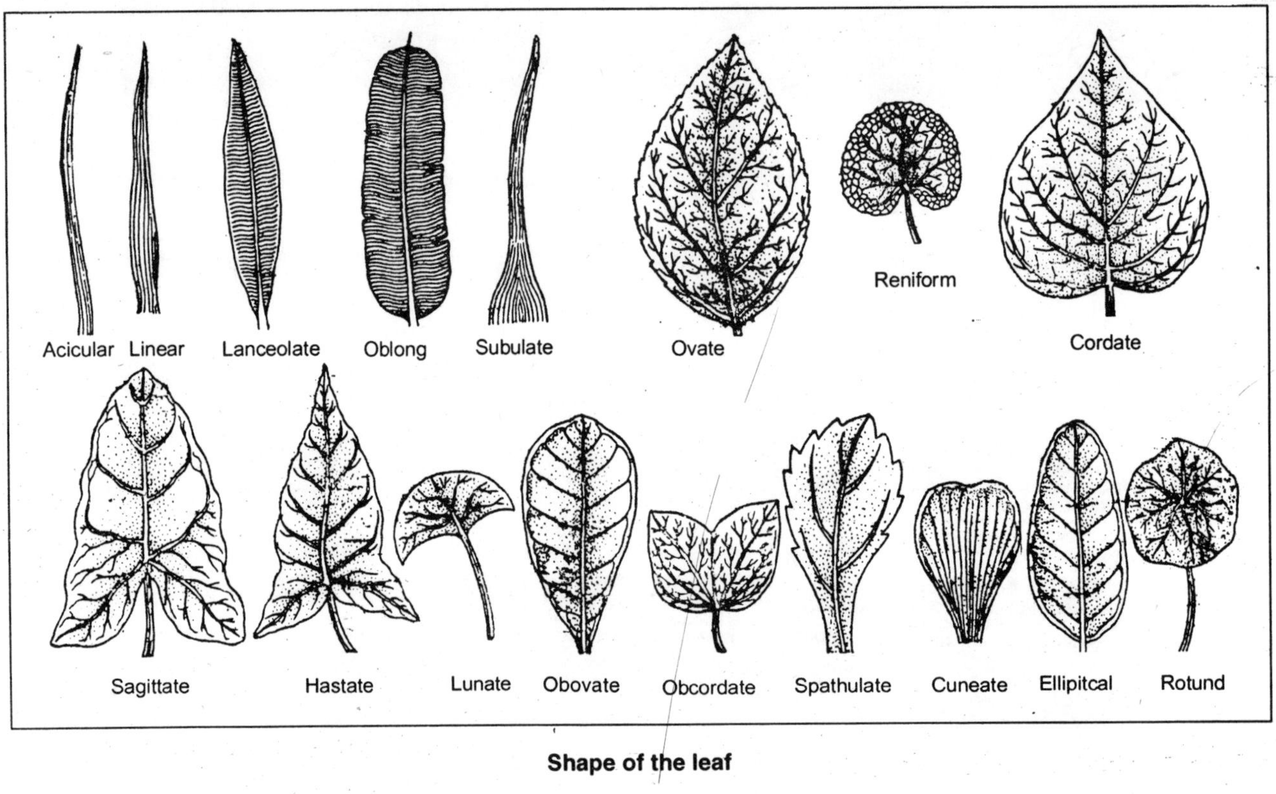

Shape of the leaf

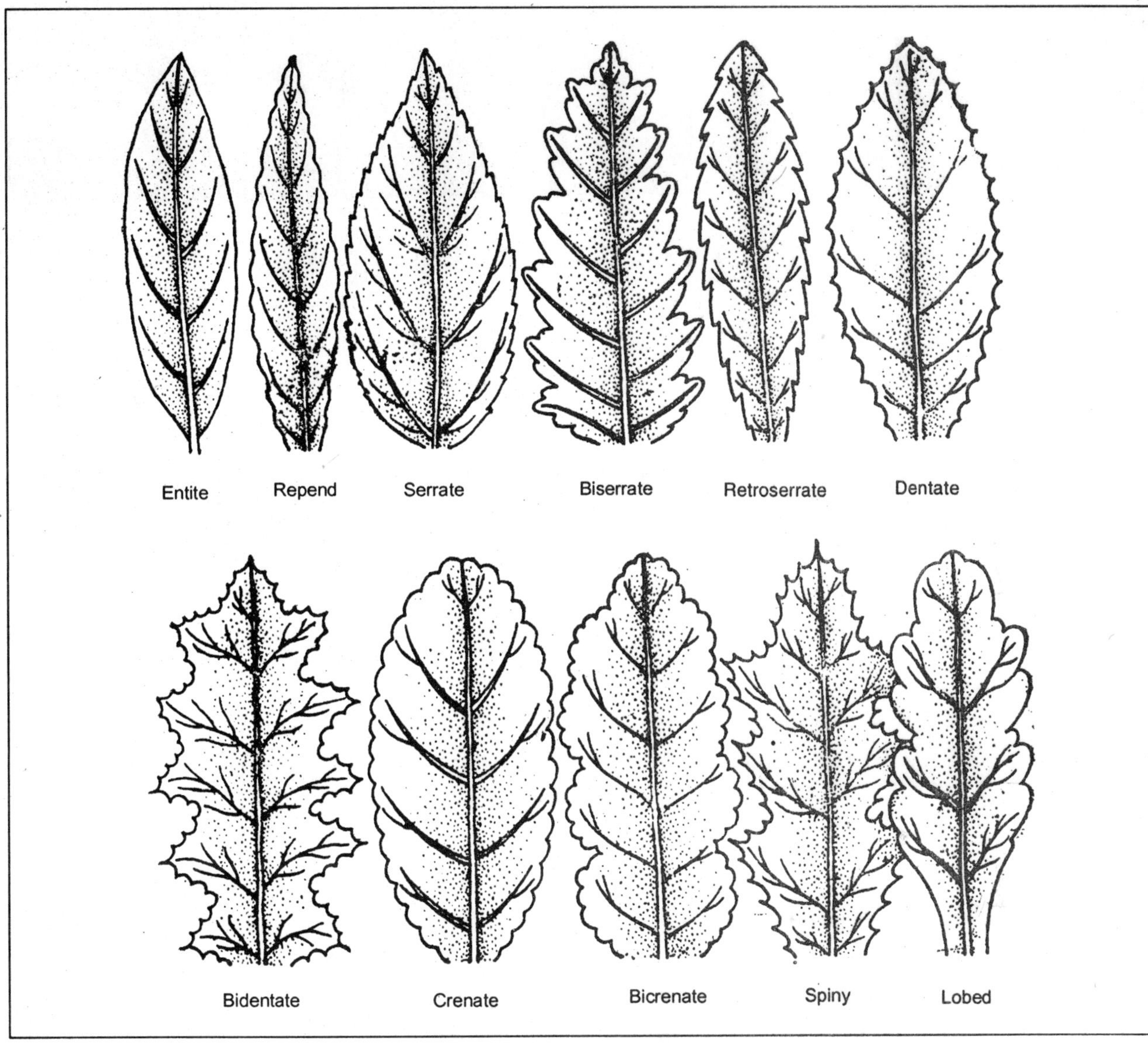

Leaf—Margin

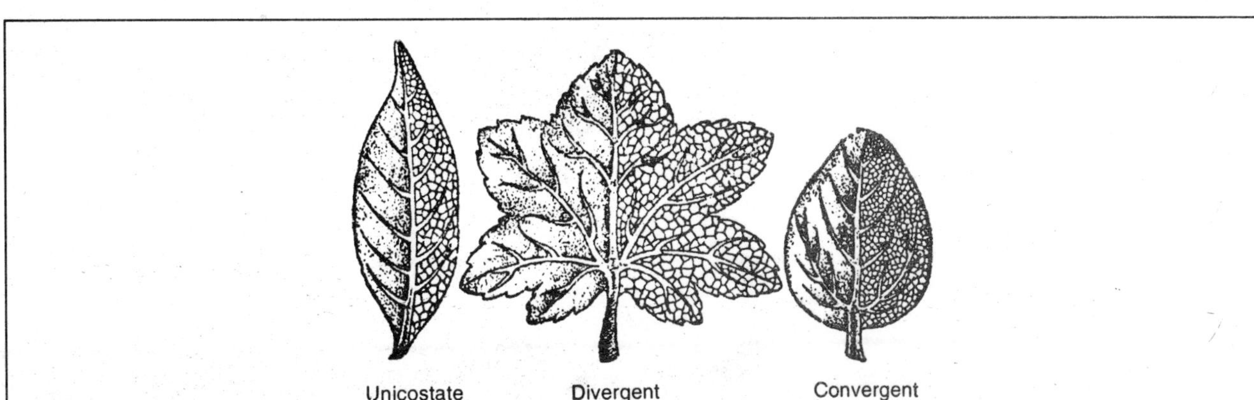

Reticulate venation

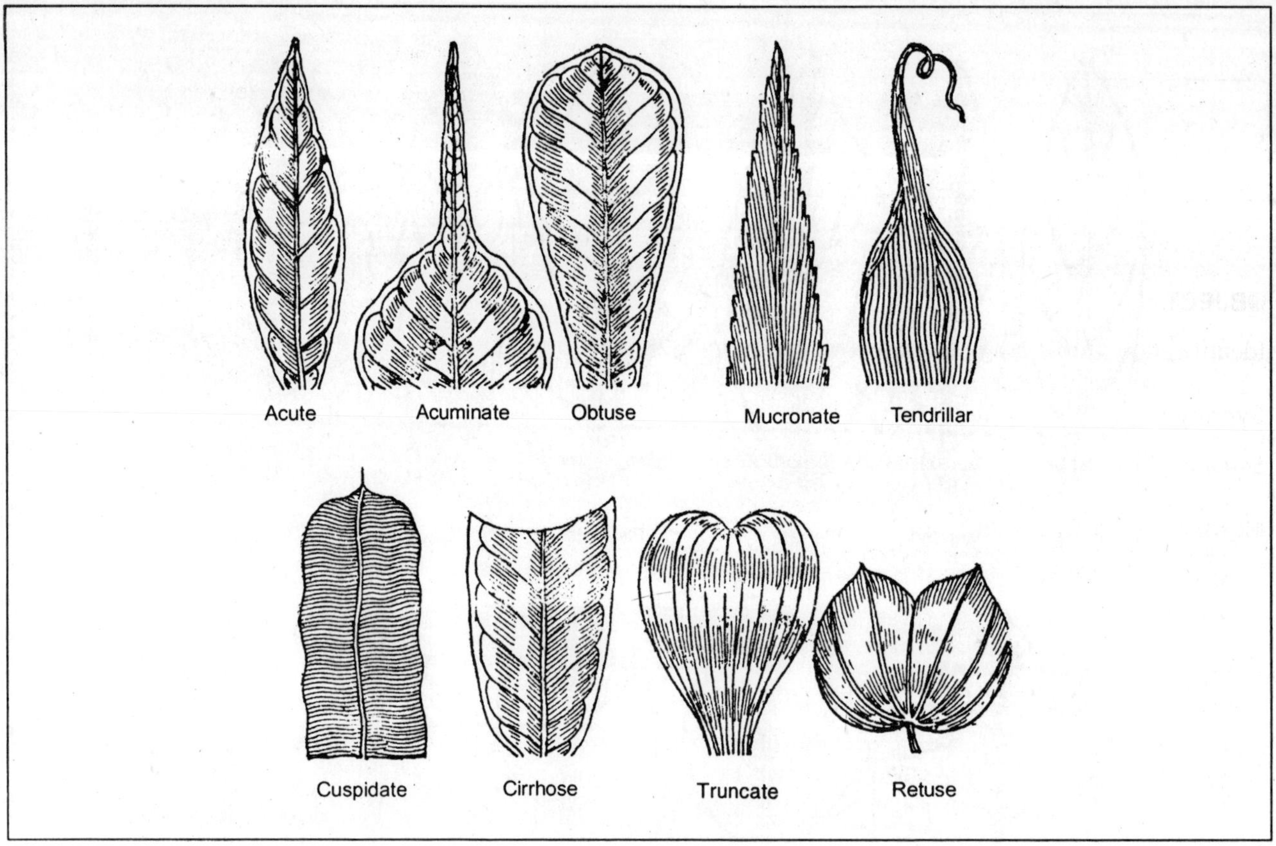

Leaf apex

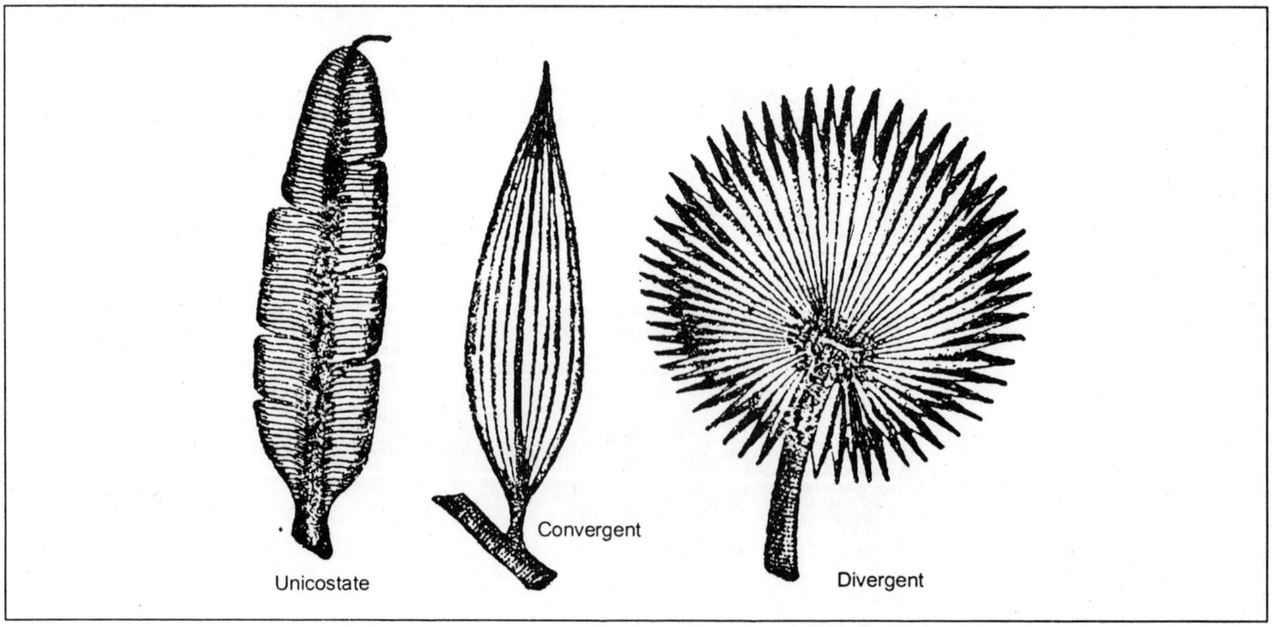

Parallel venation

Experiment 1

OBJECT

Identification of leaf drug **Senna** by study of morphological characters.

Synonyms

Sanai ki patti, Indian Senna, Tinnevelly Senna, etc.

Morphological characters

Size	2.5–6.0 cm long, up to 1 cm wide
Shape of lamina	Lanceolate
Apex of lamina	Acute–Sharp and fine
Margin of lamina	Entire
Base of lamina	Asymmetric
surface	Pubescent (hairy)
Texture of leaf	Thin, brittle
Type of leaf	Compound-pinnate

Organoleptic characters

Colour	Yellowish Green
Odour	Slight and characteristic
Taste	Mucilaginous and slightly bitter

Chemical constituents

It contains anthraquinone glycosides, i.e. sennoside A, B, C and D. It also contains kaempferol, mucilage, calcium oxalate and resin.

Use

Laxative

Biological source

The given sample of crude drug consists of dried leaflets of *Cassia angustifolia* belonging to the family Leguminosae.

Experiment 2

OBJECT

Identification of leaf drug **Digitalis** by study of morphological characters.

Synonyms

Foxglove, Fairy glove.

Morphological characters

Size	10–20 cm long, up to 4–10 cm wide
Shape of lamina	Oblong, lanceolate
Apex of lamina	Obtuse or rounded
Margin of lamina	Crenate to dentate
Base of lamina	Asymmetric
Surface	Upper pubescent (hairy) lower surface more pubescent (hairy)
Texture of leaf	Paper-like
Petiole	Winged
Venation	Pinnate, midrib prominent, lateral veins leave at an acute angle
Type of leaf	Simple

Organoleptic characters

Colour	deep green to yellowish green
Odour	Tea like
Taste	Bitter

Chemical constituents

It contains purpuria glycosides A and B primarily. It also contains digitoxin, gitoxin, gitaloxin as secondary glycosides of medicinal importance.

Use

Cordiotonic.

Biological source

The given sample of crude drug consists of dried leaves of *Digitalis purpuria* belonging to the family Scrophulariaceae.

Experiment 3

OBJECT

Identification of leaf drug **Vasaka** by study of morphological characters.

Synonyms

Adulasa, Adhatoda.

Morphological characters

Size	10–20 cm long, 3.5–6 cm wide
Shape of lamina	Ovate-lanceolate
Apex of lamina	Acuminate
Margin of lamina	Slightly crenate to entire
Base of lamina	Tapering
Surface	Glabrous (smooth) or slightly pubescent (hairy)
Texture of leaf	Thin, leathery
Venation	Pinnate, prominent midrib
Type of leaf	Simple

Organoleptic characters

Colour	Light green
Odour	Slight
Taste	Bitter

Chemical constituents

It contains alkaloids like vasicine, vasicinone, betain and vasakin.

Use

As expectorant, chronic bronchitis, asthma, etc.

Biological source

The given sample of crude drug consists of the fresh or dried leaves of *Adhatoda vasaka* belonging to the family Acanthaceae.

Experiment 4

OBJECT

Identification of leaf drug **Gymnema** by study of morphological characters.

Synonym

Gurmar.

Morphological characters

Size	3.2–5 cm long, 1.3–3.2 cm wide
Shape of lamina	Ovate, elliptic or ovate, lanceolate
Apex of lamina	Acute or shortly acuminate
Base of lamina	Rounded or cordate some time cuneate
Surface	More or less pubescent on both sides
Type of leaf	Simple opposite

Organoleptic characters

Colour	Deep green
Odour	Pleasant aromatic
Taste	Tasteless

Chemical constituents

Gymnemic acid, albumin, organic acid, pararabin, and chlorophylls, phytin, resins, tartaric acid, formic acid and butyric acid.

Use

As antidiabitic, stomachic, stimulant, diuretic, cough, etc.

Biological source

The given sample of crude drug consists of *Gymnema sylvestre* belonging to the family Ascleapidaceae.

Experiment 5

OBJECT

Identification of leaf drug **Tulsi** by study of morphological characters.

Synonym

Sacred basil.

Morphological characters

Size	2–5 cm long, 1.5–3 cm wide
Shape of lamina	Elliptical
Apex of lamina	Acute
Margin of lamina	Entire or serrate
Base of lamina	Slender
Surface	Pubescent (hairy) on both side
Texture of leaf	Thin
Venation	Pinnate

Flowers

Inflorescence	Verticillate, racemes
Calyx	Slender, pubescent, bilabiate
Corolla	Hypogynous.
Stamens	4, unequal pairs
Ovary	free, 4 lobed, style simple.

Organoleptic characters

Colour	Green
Odour	Aromatic
Taste	Aromatic

Chemical constituents

The main constituent is volatile oils, i.e. eugenol, methyl eugenol, carvacrol, caryophyllin, etc.

Use

Expectorant, diaphoretic, antiseptic, spasmolytics, antiperiodic, etc. It is also useful in bronchitis, fever, cough, cold and gastric disorder.

Biological source

The given sample of crude drug consists of *Ocimum sanctum* belonging to the family Labiatae.

Experiment 6

OBJECT

Identification of leaf drug **Belladonna** by study of morphological characters.

Synonym

Deadly night shade leaves.

Morphological characters

Size	5–25 cm long 2.5–12 cm wide
Shape of lamina	Ovate, decurrent lamina
Apex of lamina	Acuminate
Margin of lamina	Entire
Base of lamina	Acute or slightly decurrent
Surface	Glabrous
Texture of leaf	Thin
Leaf	Stalked, brittle

Organoleptic characters

Colour	Dull-green or yellowish- green

Chemical constituents

It contains alkaloids, i.e. l-hyoscyamine, atropine, apoatropine, belladonin, scopolamine, etc. It also contains volatile oils and calcium oxalate.

Use

It is anticholinergic and mydriatic agent. It is also useful in asthma and whooping cough.

Biological source

The given sample of crude drug consists of dried leaves of *Atropa belladonna* belonging to the family Solanaceae.

Experiment 7

OBJECT

Identification of leaf drug **Nim** by study of morphological characters.

Synonyms

Neem, nimba.

Morphological characters

Size	3- 6 cm long
Shape of lamina	Ovate, lanceolate
Margin of lamina	Serrate
Stipule	Existipulate
Type of leaf	Imparipinnate, alternate

Organoleptic characters

Colour	Dark green
Odour	Typical
Taste	Bitter

Chemical constituents

Nim oil contains glycerides of palmitic acid, stearic acid, linoleic acid, etc. It also contains nimbidin, nimbin, nimbidol.

Use

As antifungal and antiseptic, stimulant, wormicide

Biological source

The given sample of crude drug consists of fresh or dried leaves of *Azadirachta indica* belonging to the family Meliacea.

5

Bark

Identification of Bark Drugs

All tissues lying out side the secondary phloem, i.e. pericycle, cortex, periderm (cork cambium, cork and secondary cortex) and all dead cells external to periderm. So bark consists of the external tissue of stems or roots removed by making longitudinal and transverse incisions.

Rhytidoma

The external covering of a bark which consists of layers of dead phloem alternating with bands of cork is termed as rhytidoma.

Methods of collection

1. Felling

The fully grown tree was cut down near the ground level and barks are removed from stem and branches, e.g. cinchona.

2. Uprooting

It is the most common method of collection. The root is dug up and the barks are removed from the truck, branches and root of the 10–15 years old tree.

3. Copping

In this case the tree is allowed to grow. The stem is then cut down to within short distance from the ground and the bark is removed. The stools are allowed to grow again and the bark is stripped from them.

Shape of pieces

Depending on the type of incisions made to the bark, the nature and extent of the shrinkage which occurs during drying the bark, are characterized by the following features.

(a) Flats

When finished bark consists of flat pieces, e.g. cinchona.

(b) Curved

When only slightly concave on the inside.

(c) Re-curved

When concavity is on the out side.

(d) Channelled

When the curvature on the inside is so great to form channel.

(e) Quill

When the curvature is so deep that the one edge overlaps the other.

(f) Double Quill

When each edge is rolled independently in to a quill.

(g) Compound quill

When quills are packed one inside the other, e.g. cinnamon.

CHARACTERS OF THE OUTER SURFACE

(a) Smooth

When the cork is evenly developed.

(b) Scaly

When rhytidoma is present.

(c) Exfoliates

The corky layer frequently flakes off.

(d) Cracks and fissures

It happens owing to the lack of elasticity in the dead tissue.

(e) Wrinkles

The wrinkles appears due to shrinkage of the softer tissue.

(f) Furrows

When the troughs between the wrinkles are very wide.

Characters of inner surface

- **(a) Striations:** Due to formation of parallel longitudinal ridges.
- **(b) Corrugations:** The longitudinal shrinkage produces parallel transverse wrinkles.

Fracture

The nature of exposed surfaces of a transversely broken bark is called fracture.

(a) Short: The surfaces are smooth.

(b) Granular: The surfaces exhibit small rounded structures.

(c) Splintery: When jagged projecting points are formed.

(d) Fibrous: When the surface consists of fine fibrous threads.

(e) Laminated: When fractured region breaks in to tangentially arranged layers.

Experiment 8

OBJECT

Identification of Bark drug **Arjuna** by study of morphological characters.

Synonyms

Arjun, Anjan.

Morphological characters

Size	2–4 cm long, 10 mm wide and 0.3–1 cm in thickness.
Outer surface	Smooth and gray colour.
Inner surface	Striated and brown.
Fractures	Short and fibrous.

Organoleptic characters

Colour outer surface	Gray
Colour inner surface	Brown
Odour	Odourless
Taste	Astringent

Chemical constituents

It contains tannins, triterpenoid, saponins, arjunine, arjunetin, arjunolic acid, sugar, calcium salts, essential oil and traces of aluminium and magnesium salts.

Use

Cardiotonic, astringent, diuretic, febrifuge, etc.

Biological source

The given sample of crude drug consists of dried bark of *Terminalia arjuna* belonging to the family Combretaceae.

Experiment 9

OBJECT

Identification of Bark drug **Ashok** by study of morphological characters.

Synonym

Asoka.

Morphological characters

Size	40 cm long, 4–6 mm wide and 5–8 mm thick.
Shape	Channelled.
Outer surface	Smooth with circular lenticels or transversely ridged or cracked.
Inner surface	Smooth and longitudinally striated.
Fractures	Short and fibrous.

Organoleptic characters

Colour outer surface	Yellowish to gray
Colour inner surface	Reddish brown
Odour	Odourless
Taste	Astringent and bitter

Chemical constituents

It contains tannins, catechol, sterol, phlobaphenes, organic calcium compound and ketosterol.

Use

Astringent and uterine tonic.

Biological source

The given sample of crude drug consists of dried bark of *Saraca indica*, belonging to the family Leguminosae.

Experiment 10

OBJECT

Identification of Bark drug **Cinchona** by study of morphological characters.

Morphological characters

Size	Up to 30 cm long, diameter 15–20 mm and thickness 2–8 mm.
Shape	Compound quill.
Outer surface	Rough due to presence of cracks, wrinkles and often bears epiphytes such as lichens.
Inner surface	Longitudinal striations.
Fractures	Short and fibrous.
Root bark	Channelled, twisted, outer surface-scaly, inner surface-striated.

Organoleptic characters

Colour outer surface	Greyish green
Colour inner surface	Reddish brown
Odour	Odourless
Taste	Bitter or more less astringent

Chemical constituents

It contains alkaloids like quinine, quinidine, cinchonine and cinchonidine. Other constituents are quinovin, oxidase, calcium oxalate and starch.

Use

Antimalarial and antipyretic. It is used to treat cardiac arrhythmias.

Biological source

The given sample of crude drug consists of root or stem bark of *Cinchona calisaya* and other species, belonging to the family Rubiaceae.

Experiment 11

OBJECT

Identification of bark drug **Cinnamon** by study of morphological characters.

Morphological characters

Size	Up to 100 cm long, diameter 6–10 mm thickness 0.5 mm.
Shape	Single or double compound quill.
Outer surface	Longitudinal wavy lines and occasional scars and holes.
Inner surface	Longitudinal striations.
Fractures	Short, splintery.

Organoleptic characters

Colour outer surface	Yellowish brown
Colour inner surface	Dark green
Odour	Aromatic
Taste	Warm sweet

Chemical constituents

Volatile oil consists of eugenol, pinene, phellandrene, caryophyllene and cinnamyl acetate. It also contains mucilage, calcium oxalate, sugar starch and phlobatannin.

Use

Carminative, Stomachic.

Biological source

The given sample of crude drug consists of dried bark of *Cinnamomum zeylanicum* belonging to the family Lauraceae.

6

Flower

Identification of Flower Drugs

A flower is modified condensed shoot specialized to carry out sexual reproduction in higher plants.

Bract

A small leaf like structure which arises at the axil. It is situated at the base of the pedicel.

(a) *Bracteate:* Bract present. (b) *Ebracteate:* Bract absent.

Bracteole

A small leaf like structures are present in the middle of pedicel.

(a) *Bracteolate:* Bracteole present. (b) *Ebracteolate:* Bracteole absent.

Pedicellate

Pedicel present.

Sessile

Pedicel absent.

Type of flower

Flower may be hermaphrodite or unisexual.

Whorls of flower

A flower consists of four whorls, i.e. calyx, corolla, androecium and gynoecium. Out of which calyx and corolla are non essential or helping whorls. Androecium and gynoecium are fertile or essential whorls.

Calyx

It is the outermost whorl. The individual unit is called sepal. In bud condition it encloses the inner part of the flower.

Corolla

The individual unit is called petal. Petals are the large coloured attractive part of the flower.

Androecium

It is the male part of the flower. The individual unit is called stamen. Each stamen consists of the anther and filament.

Gynoecium (Pistil)

It is a female part of the flower and individual unit is called carpel. Each carpel consists of ovary, stigma and style. The oval structures are found in the ovary is called ovules which forms seeds after fertilization.

Experiment 12

OBJECT

Identification of flower drug **Clove** by study of morphological characters.

Synonym

Lavang.

Morphological characters

Size	16–20 mm long.
Origin	Buds.
Type of Inflorescences	Mixed (racemes of cymes in clove).
Receptacle (thalamus)	Stalk of the ovary
Calyx	4 no. of sepals, thick walled, spreading.
Corolla	4 no. of petals.
Androecium	Indefinite no. of stamens, tetradelphous. The anthers are entrose.
Gynoecium	Inferior, the erect central and cylindrical style and bilocular ovary.
Ovules	Numerous no. in each locules,.
Special feature	*Hypanthium:* It is lower solid stalk which is sub cylindrical, slightly flattened and tapering below about 10–13 mm long, 4 mm wide and 2 mm thick. *Crown:* It consists of calyx, corolla, stamen and style.

Organoleptic characters

Colour outer surface	Reddish brown, rough surface.
Odour	Strong, spicy and aromatic.
Taste	Pungent and aromatic.

Chemical constituents

It contains volatile oils, tannins, triterpenic acid, vanillin, gum and resin. The volatile constituents are eugenol, acetyl eugenol, methyl amyl euginol, and caryophyllenes. methyl furfural and carbinol.

Use

It is used in dyspepsia, flatulence, toothache and as flavouring agent.

Biological source

The given sample of crude drug consists of flower bud of *Eugenia carryophyllus*, belonging to the family Myrtaceae.

Experiment 13

OBJECT

Identification of flower drug **Pyrethrum** by study of morphological characters.

Morphological characters

Size	The closed heads flowers are nearly 6–9 mm in diameter and open heads are 9–12 mm in diameter.
Peduncle	It is short striated longitudinally.
Receptacle	It is 4–8 mm in diameter, flat and without paleae. It is surrounded by an involucre of 2 or 3 rows of bracts which are hairy and lanceolate with a membranous margin.

The flower of pyrethrum is of two types

Ray florets (ligulate)	It is simple row of 15–23 in number.
Calyx	Tubular, membranous.
Corolla	White about 16 mm long with three rounded apical teeth, the central one being often more or less suppressed.
Gynoecium	Inferior ovary, about 5 mm long and 5 ribbed.
Style	Filiform, stigma bifid.

Discflorets (Tubular)

It is of 200–300 in numbers, each with a yellow, tubular, corolla and five epipetalous stamens. Gynoecium and calyx are as in ray floret.

Organoleptic characters

Odour	Aromatic
Taste	Bitter, acrid

Chemical constituents

It contains pyrethrin I and II, cinarin I and II, Jasmolin I and II, volatile oil, sesquiterpenes lactones, triterpenoid oil pyrethrol.

Use

Used as a contact poison for insects in form of powder of crude drug.

Biological source

The given sample of crude drug consists of flower heads of *Chrysanthemum cinerariaefolium* belonging to the family Compositae.

7

Fruit

Identification of Fruit Drugs

The enlarged and mature single ovary after fertilization enclosing seeds is called fruit.

Classification—3 types

(A) Simple fruit: It is formed from a carpel or from a syncarpous gynoecium.

- (A.1) Dry fruit
  - (a) Dehiscent
  - (b) Indehiscent
  - (c) Schizocarpic
    - (c.1) Lomentum
    - (c.2) Cremocarp
    - (c.3) Regma
- (A.2) Fleshy fruit

(B) Aggregate fruit: It is formed from an apocarpous gynoecium.

(C) Compound fruit: It is formed from an inflorescence.

Cremocarpic

All fruits belong to umbelliferae family are of cremocarpic fruit. The cremocarp is a type of schizocarpic fruit which is simple dry indehiscent fruit. The cremocarpic fruits split into two identical parts called **mericarps**. The central stalk which joins the mericarps is called **carpophore**. Stylopod is a disc like nectary structure which contain style and calyx at the apex of mericarp. Each mericarp has two surfaces. The outer one is called dorsal while the inner one is known as ventral or commissural surface.

The wavy inconspicuous ridges are found on the surface of mericarp. Similarly the straight longitudinal prominent ridges are called **secondary ridges** on the surface of mericarp. **Vittae** is the schizogenous ducts extending through the mesocarp from base to apex containing volatile oils. The number and the position of these vittae are often characteristics of individual fruit.

Experiment 14

OBJECT

Identification of fruit drug **Amla** by study of morphological characters.

Synonym

Indian goose berry.

Morphological characters

Class	Drupes fleshy.
Size, Shape	1.5–2.5 cm in diameter, oval or globose.
Dehiscence	Indehiscent
Pericarp	The surface bears numerous furrows which divides the fruit in six lobes. The surface is smooth and shiny.
Depression	It is formed due to removal of peduncle at one end.
Endocarp	Hard.

Organoleptic characters

Colour	Green to light yellow.
Odour	Odourless.
Taste	Sour and astringent.

Chemical constituents

The main chemical constituent is vitamin C. It also contains pectin, minerals like Fe, P, Ca, etc. tannins, glucose, gallic acid and ellagic acid.

Use

As source of vitamin C, diuretic, laxative. It is useful in anaemia, jaundice, dyspepsia and diabetes.

Biological source

The given sample of crude drug consists of fresh or dried fruits of *Emblica officinalis* belonging to the family Euphorbiaceae.

Experiment 15

OBJECT

Identification of fruit drug **Coriander** by study of morphological characters.

Synonym

Dhaniya.

Morphological characters

Class	Entire cremocarp.
Size, Shape	3–5 mm in diameter, sub-spherical.
Mericarp	Two mericarps are united by their margins.
Pericarp	Each mericarp has five wavy inconspicuous primary ridges and four straight more prominent secondary ridges.
Vittae	Each mericarp has two vittae on the commissural surface. In addition to these. The young ovary contains vittae on the dorsal surface as the fruit ripens these become compressed and break down in to tangentially elongated cavities.
Stylopod	Present at the apex of the fruit.
Seed	Coelospermous.

Organoleptic characters

Colour	Yellowish brown
Odour	Aromatic
Taste	Spicy

Chemical constituents

The chief volatile constituents are d-linalol, others are pinene, geraniol, borneol, dipentone, phellandrine, etc. It also contains fixed oil, malic acid, tannin, mucilage, etc.

Use

Aromatic, carminative, stomachic and stimulant.

Biological source

The given sample of crude drug consists of dried ripe fruits of *Coriandrum sativum* belonging to the family Umbelliferae.

Experiment 16

OBJECT

Identification of fruit drug **Caraway** by study of morphological characters.

Synonym

Zira

Morphological characters

Condition	Mericarps without pedicels.
Size, Shape	4–7 mm long, 1 mm wide, slightly curve, smooth and tapering at both ends.
Pericarp	Primary ridges–5 in number.
Vittae	Four vittae on dorsal surface and two on commissural surface.
Stylopod	Present at the apex of the fruit.

Organoleptic characters

Colour	Brown.
Odour	Aromatic, spicy.
Taste	Characteristic.

Chemical constituents

It contains volatile oils, fixed oil, protein, calcium oxalate, resins, tannins and mucilage. The volatile constituents are carvone, dihydrocarvone, limonene, carveol, etc.

Use

Aromatic, carminative, stomachic and lactagogue.

Biological source

The given sample of crude drug consists of dried ripe fruits of *Carum carvi* belonging to the family Umbelliferae.

Experiment 17

OBJECT

Identification of fruit drug **Cardamom** by study of morphological characters.

Synonym

Ilayachi.

Morphological characters

Condition	The fruit develop from inferior capsule.
Size, shape	1–2 cm long, ovoid and more or less three sided with rounded angles.
Base	Rounded and bears the remains of the pedicel.
Apex	Slight projection consisting of remains of perianth.
Surface	Longitudinally striated.
Placentation	Axile.
Seed	It develops from anatropous ovules. Each capsules contains 5–12 seeds. Shape and size — irregularly ovoid with flattened faces and rounded angles, 3 mm long.
Aril	A colour less membranous structure around the seeds which become thicker and oily in mature seeds.
Surface	It bears transverse wrinkles and groove is called raphae. The hilum is situated at the base.
Testa	Dark reddish brown.
Perisperm	Starchy.
Endosperm	Small and yellowish.
Embryo	Cylindrical small containing aleuron grains.

Organoleptic characters

Odour	Aromatic
Taste	Agreeable pungent

Chemical constituents

Volatile oils, fixed oil, starch, calcium oxalate and vitamin B_1. The volatile oils contains cineole, borneol, terpeniol, limonene, terpine, dipentene, etc.

Use

Aromatic, carminative, diuretic and flavouring agent.

Biological source

The given sample of crude drug consists of dried ripe capsule and seeds of *Elettaria cardamomum* belonging to the family Zingiberaceae.

Experiment 18

OBJECT

Identification of fruit drug **Ajowan** by study of morphological characters.

Morphological characters

Condition	Mericarp separate.
Size, Shape	2 mm long, 1.5 mm wide, ovoid.
Primary ridges	5 in number, pale in colour.
Vittae	Six in number in each mericarp.

Organoleptic characters

Colour	Greenish brown.
Odour	Odour of thymol.
Taste	Spicy.

Chemical constituents

The chief volatile constituent is thymol. It also contains protein and tannin.

Use

Aromatic, carminative and flavouring agent. It is also a source of thymol.

Biological source

The given sample of crude drug consists of dried ripe fruits of *Trachyspermum ammi* of the family Umbelliferae.

Experiment 19

OBJECT

Identification of fruit drug **Black pepper** by study of morphological characters.

Synonyms

Gol mirch, kali mirch.

Morphological characters

Size, shape	4-5 mm in diameter, globular.
Pericarp	Thin and encloses a single seed with a hollow centre.
Surface	Coated with deep set wrinkles.

Organoleptic characters

Colour	Deep brown to black.
Odour	Aromatic.
Taste	Spicy.

Chemical constituents

It contains the alkaloids piperine, piperidine, piperettine, etc. The volatile oils are phellandrene, caryophyllene, piperonal, dihydrocarveol, α and β pinenes. It also contains starch, thiamine, riboflavin, nicotinic acid, ascorbic acid and carotene.

Use

Aromatic, carminative and stimulant. Externally as rubifacient.

Biological source

The given sample of crude drug consists of dried unripe fruits of *Piper nigrum* of the family Piperaceae.

Experiment 20

OBJECT

Identification of fruit drug **Orange peel** by study of morphological characters.

Synonym

Fructus aurantii.

Morphological characters

Orange peel	The fresh orange peel is cut from the orange when required for use. It is outermost part of pericarp. The dried peel is hard and brittle.
Size	2–6 mm thick, 6–12 mm wide.
Outer surface	It is dark orange red, rough due to raising over oil glands. It contains small pits and reticulate ridges.
Inner surface	Yellowish white.
Fracture	Hard and short.

Organoleptic characters

Odour	Aromatic
Taste	Aromatic and bitter

Chemical constituents

It contains volatile oils, vitamin C, hesperidine, neohesperidine, aurantiamarin, resin, gum and tannin.

Use

Aromatic, carminative and flavouring agent.

Biological source

The given sample of crude drug consists of dried rind of nearly ripe fruit of *Citrum aurantium* and other species of the family Rutaceae.

Experiment 21

OBJECT

Identification of fruit drug **Lemon peel** by study of morphological characters.

Synonym

Fructus limonis.

Morphological characters

Lemon peel	The fresh lemon peel is the outer part of the pericarp.
Size	20 cm long, 1.5 cm wide, 2–3 mm thick.
Shape	Spiral, strips.
Outer surface	Yellow to yellowish brown, rough.
Inner surface	Pithy and white.

Organoleptic characters

Odour	Strong and aromatic.
Taste	Aromatic and bitter.

Chemical constituents

It contains volatile oils, vitamin B and C, hesperidine, mucilage, pectin, calcium oxalate and flavone glycosides.

Use

Aromatic, carminative and flavouring agent.

Biological source

The given sample of crude drug consists of dried /fresh lemon peel from the fresh ripe fruit of *Citrus lemon* of the family Rutaceae.

Experiment 22

OBJECT

Identification of fruit drug **Bahera** by study of morphological characters.

Synonym

Bahira.

Morphological characters

Type of fruit	Drupe.
Size	1.3–2.5 cm in diameter.
Shape	Ovoid.
Outer surface	5 well defined longitudinal ridges are present a long with irregular wrinkles. The scar of pedicel is found at one end of the fruit.
Texture	Very hard.

Organoleptic characters

Colour	Broken surface is yellow.
Odour	Odourless.
Taste	Astringent.

Chemical constituents

It contains tannins, fixed oils, mannitol, rhamnose, fructose, glucose, β sitosterol, etc.

Use

It is used in dysentery, dyspepsia, dropsy, leprosy and constipation.

Biological source

The given sample of crude drug consists of dried ripe fruit of *Terminalia belerica* of the family Combretaceae.

Experiment 23

OBJECT

Identification of fruit drug **Gokhru** by study of morphological characters.

Morphological characters

Chhota gokhru

Size	1–1.2 cm in diameter.
Shape	Globose.
Outer surface	Each fruit contains five woody spiny cocci and each coccus bears to sharp pointed spines directed towards the apex. The other spines are directed downwards.

Bara gokhru

Size	2 cm long.
Shape	Pyramid ovoidal and tapering at the base and apex.
Surface	Each fruit has four spines and it tapers in to hollow cylindrical tube toward both ends.

Chemical constituents

It contains saponine glycoside, flavone glycoside, alkaloid, fixed oil, resin, potassium nitrate, mucilage and volatile oil.

Use

As diuretic, aphrodisiac. It is given in nocturnal emission, dysuria, impotency, gout, kidney disease and calculus affections.

Biological source

The given sample of chhota gokhru consists of dried ripe fruit of *Tribulus terrestris* of the family Zygophyllaceae.

The given sample of Bara gokhru consists of dried ripe fruit of *Pedalium murex* of the family Pedaliaceae.

8

Seed

Identification of Seed Drugs

Seed is fertilized mature ovule which contains an embryo.

Seed coat

It is an outer covering of the seed which develop from the integuments from the ovules.

Testa and Tegmen

The outer coat is called testa and the inner layer is called tegmen. The testa is hard where as tegmen is thin and membranous.

Hilum

It is the mark of attachment with the stalk on outer surface of the seed.

Mycropyle

A small hole in the ovule is being left through which the pollen tube may pass on it way to the embryosac.

Nucellus

A mass of parenchymatous tissue of the ovule is called nucellus.

Perisperm

In some seed like cardamom and pepper, the nucellus develops to form a storage tissue called perisperm.

Funicle

The part of ovule which joins with placenta. The ovule without funicle is called sessile ovule.

Raphe

It is short ridge like structures which serves as path from funicle to chalaza. Chalaza is the base of the ovule.

Integuments

It is one or two layer around the nucellus. The number of integuments are the characteristics of a particular family.

Embryo

The embryo is differentiated in to radicle, plumule and cotyledons. The radicle gives rise to primary root where as plumule gives rise to aerial shoot.

Albuminous and exalbuminous seeds

Albuminous

The seeds which store food materials in endosperm, e.g. castor, wheat.

Exalbuminous

The seeds which store food materials in their cotyledons, e.g. almond, ground nut, etc.

Forms of ovules

1. Orthotropus

Funicle, chalaza and micropyle of a ovule are situated in a straight line, e.g. polygonace, piperaceae.

2. Antropous

The ovule is completely inverted. The nucellus is parallel to funicle. The micropyle comes near to hilum. The degree of curvature 180°.

3. Hemitropous ovule

It is intermediate between orthotropus and antropous, i.e. at right angle to funicle. The micropyle–chalaza line is horizontal and placed at 90° to the line of funicle.

4. Campylotropous

The body of ovule becomes curved so that the micropyle and chalaza come to line on either side of the funicle. The raphe is not formed.

5. Amphitropous

The ovule curved to form horseshoe shaped.

6. Circinotropous

The ovule is straight with micropyle facing upwards. The funicle is elongated and coiled. It completely encircles the ovule.

Morphology of seeds consists of the following characters

1. *Physical character:* Shape, dimension, hardness, etc.
2. *Seed coat:* Number, marking, hilum, raphe, aril, etc.
3. *Perisperm:* Present or absent, nature of reserves.
4. *Endosperm:* Present or absent nature of reserve.
5. *Embryo*
   (a) Position, shape, dimensions.
   (b) Cotyledons — colour, outline and venation.
   (c) Radicle.
   (d) Odour and taste.
   (e) Others.

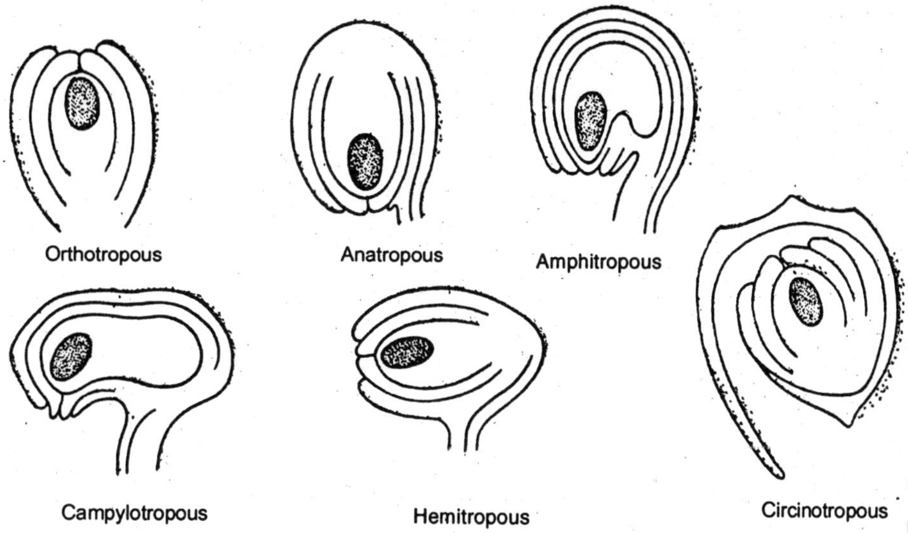
Orthotropous
Anatropous
Amphitropous
Campylotropous
Hemitropous
Circinotropous

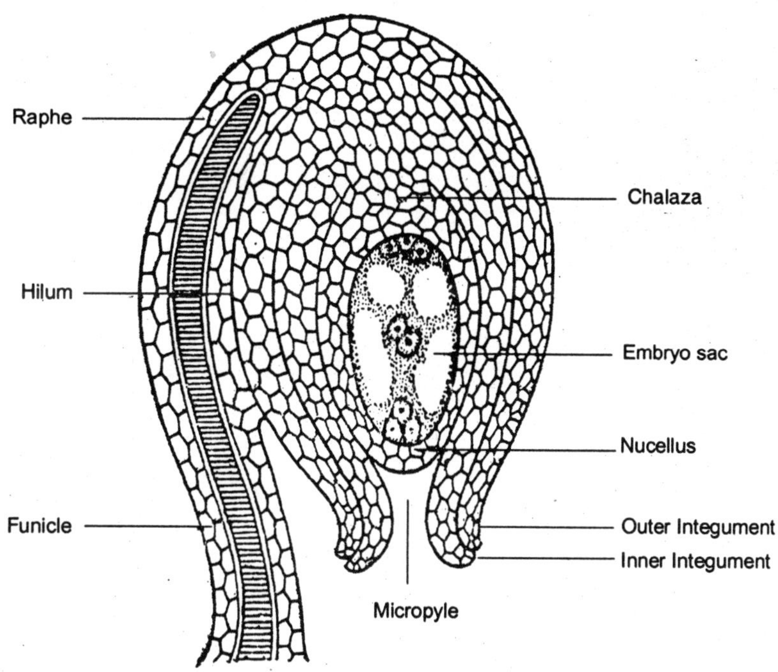
Raphe
Chalaza
Hilum
Embryo sac
Nucellus
Funicle
Outer Integument
Inner Integument
Micropyle

L.S. of ovule

Experiment 24

OBJECT

Identification of seed drug **Isphagula** by study of morphological characters.

Synonyms

Isabgol, isapgol.

Morphological characters

Size, shape	1.8–3.3 mm long, 1–1.7 mm wide, boat shaped or oval.
Seed coats	Convex surface brown oval spot is present; concave surface–hilum covered with thin whitish membrane.
Embryo	Containing cotyledon.
Other characters	When soaked in water, the seed coat swells and the seeds become surrounded with a transparent colourless mucilage.

Organoleptic characters

Colour	Pale greyish brown
Odour	Odourless
Taste	Mucilaginous

Chemical constituents

Main constituent is mucilage. It also contains fixed oil, protein and amino acid.

Use

Laxative and demulscent.

Biological source

The given sample of crude drug consists of dried seed of *Plantago ovata* belonging to the family Plataginaceae.

Experiment 25

OBJECT

Identification of seed drug **Nux vomica** seed by study of morphological characters.

Synonym

Kuchla.

Morphological characters

Size, shape	10–30 mm in diameter, 3–5 mm thick, disc shaped, flat.
Margin	Rounded.
Hilium and micropyle	Hilum is in the centre of flat surface. Micropyle is situated at one point of the margin.
Outer surface	It is covered with silky hairs radiating from the centre.
Endosperm	Horny about 2 mm thick.
Embryo	It is situated at micropyle end and whitish in colour. It contains cylindrical radicle and cotyledons.

Organoleptic characters

Colour	Outer surface gray to greenish gray.
Odour	Odourless.
Taste	Bitter and poisonous.

Chemical constituents

It consists of alkaloids, i.e. strychnine, brucine, vomicine, etc. loganin glycoside, fixed oil, proteins and aleurone grains.

Use

Bitter tonic and dyspepsia.

Biological source

The given sample of crude drug consists of dried ripe seeds of *Strychnos nux vomica* belonging to the family Loganiaceae.

Experiment 26

OBJECT

Identification of seed drug **Linseed** by study of morphological characters.

Synonyms

Alsi, linum.

Morphological characters

Size, shape	4–6 mm in long, 2–3 mm wide 1.5 mm thick, elongated, ovate and flattened.
Seed coat	Hilum is a slight hollow, close to the pointed end.
Micropyle	It is present close to hilum.
Testa	Thin, dark brown in colour, finely pitted, smooth and shining.
Endosperm	Narrow endosperm surrounding the embryo.
Embryo	Straight containing two large plano-convex cotyledons and radicle directed towards the hiler end.
Raphe	It extends as yellowish line from hilum to distal end of the seed.

Organoleptic characters

Colour	Brown
Odour	Odourless
Taste	Mucilaginous

Chemical constituents

It consists of fixed oil, mucilage, protein, linamarin and linase.

Use

Demulcent, poultice and bulk laxative.

Biological source

The given sample of crude drug consists of dried ripe seeds of *Linum usitatissimum* belonging to the family Linaceae.

Experiment 27

OBJECT

Identification of seed drug **Nutmeg** by study of morphological characters.

Synonyms

Jalphal, Jayepatri.

Morphological characters

Size, shape	20–35 mm long, 15–28 mm wide, ovoid.
Hilum and micropyle	They are present near the projection. The hilum is surrounded by a raised ring. The raphe joins the hilum with chalaza which is situated at the other end.
Outer surface	Outer surface is marked with small furrows. At one end there is small projection.
Perisperm	It is found in form of a thin layer of the outer region of the kernel.
Endosperm	It forms bulk of the nutmeg.
Embryo	It lies in a small cavity in the endosperm and its cotyledons gradually grow up in to the endosperm. The radicle is present in form of circular depression.

Organoleptic characters

Colour	The kernel is greyish brown.
Odour	Strong and aromatic.
Taste	Pungent and slightly bitter.

Chemical constituents

It contains volatile oil, starch, protein, phytosterin, amylodextrin and colouring matter. The volatile constituents are myristicin, elemicin, linalool, borneol, pinenes, camphene, dipentene, safrol, eugenol and iso-eugenol.

Use

Carminative, astringent, aphrodisiac and stomachic.

Biological source

The given sample of crude drug consists of dried ripe seeds of *Myristica fragrans* belonging to the family Myristicaceae.

Experiment 28

OBJECT

Identification of seed drug **Colchicum** by study of morphological characters.

Morphological characters

Size, shape	2–3 mm in diameter, ovoid or globular.
Hilum	It is situated at one end of the seed.
Outer surface	Pitted and very hard.
Beak	The other end is beaked.
Endosperm	Hard and oily
Embryo	It is found at the opposite side of the hilum.

Organoleptic characters

Odour	Odourless
Taste	Bitter

Chemical constituents

It contains alkaloids colchicines, demecolcine, etc. It also contains starch and colchico resin.

Use

Gout, rheumatism, myeloid and leukaemia.

Biological source

The given sample of crude drug consists of dried ripe seeds of *Colchicum autumnale* belonging to the family Liliaceae.

9

Root and Rhizome

Identification of Root and Rhizome Drugs

Root

It is non green under ground descending portion of the plant axis without nodes and internodes. There are two major type of roots, i.e. taproot and adventitious root.

Rhizome

It is a under ground modification of stem. Most of the rhizomes are fleshy and store reserve food materials. They are differentiated in to nodes and internodes.

The following features are taken in consideration for morphological study of root and rhizome.

1. Shape
2. Branching
3. Direction of growth
4. Surface characters
5. Condition
6. Types

Experiment 29

OBJECT

Identification of root drug **Aswagandha** by morphological characters.

Synonym

Withania root.

Morphological characters

Type	Tuberous root.
Size, shape	5–12 mm thick, conical.
Outer surface	It is longitudinally wrinkled.
Condition	Straight, unbranched.
Fracture	Short.

Organoleptic characters

Colour	Buff to greyish yellow.
Odour	Characteristic.
Taste	Bitter.

Chemical constituents

It mainly contains alkaloids and withanolides such as withaferin–A. Alkaloids–tropine, pseudo tropine, hygrine, isopelletierine, cuscohygrine, etc.

Use

Aphrodisiac, tonic, diuretic, narcotic, abortifacient. It is also useful in asthma, bronchintis, tuberculosis and leucorrhoea.

Biological source

The given sample of crude drug consists of dried root of *Withania somnifera* belonging to the family Solanaceae.

Experiment 30

OBJECT

Identification of root drug **Aconite** by morphological characters.

Synonym

Radix aconite.

Morphological characters

Type	Fusiform, tuberous root.
Size, shape	4–10 cm long, 1–3 cm in diameter, conical and tapering below.
Outer surface	Slightly twisted, longitudinally ridged, apical buds at the apex.
Fractured surface	Starchy.
Fracture	Short.

Organoleptic characters

Colour	Brown to dark brown.
Odour	Slight.
Taste	Initially slightly sweetish, then bitter and after an interval a sensation of numbness develops.

Chemical constituents

It contains terpinoid, alkaloids like aconitine, napelline, neoline, ephedrine, aconine, etc.

Use

It is used externally in treatment of neuralgia, rheumatism and inflammation.

Biological source

The given sample of crude drug consists of dried root of *Aconitum napellus* belonging to the family Ranunculaceae.

Experiment 31

OBJECT

Identification of rhizome drug **Ginger** by morphological characters.

Synonyms

Zingiber, Saunth

Morphological characters

Type	Rhizome
Size, shape	5–15 cm long, 3–6 cm in wide, 1–1.5 cm thick, laterally compressed, the apex of each branch a depressed scar or bud.
Outer surface	Longitudinally striations and occasional loose fibres.
Fractured surface	Cortex, endodermis and stele.
Fracture	Short and fibrous.

Organoleptic characters

Colour	Buff.
Odour	Agreeable and aromatic.
Taste	Pungent.

Chemical constituents

Volatile oils: Phellandrene, camphene, pinenes, cumene, myrcene, limonene, cineole, borneol, linalollol, zingiberene, zingerone, etc. Other constituents are resinous substances, starch, protein, sugar, etc.

Use

Flavouring agent, carminative and aromatic. It is used in sore throat, asthma, dyspepsia, cold, cough, etc.

Biological source

The given sample of crude drug consists of dried rhizome of *Zingiber officinale* belonging to the family Zingiberaceae.

Experiment 32

OBJECT

Identification of root drug **Turmeric** by morphological characters.

Synonym

Haldi, curcuma.

Morphological characters

Type	Rhizome with lateral branches, it is found in the form of 'fingers' tapering on both ends.
Size	4–7 cm long, 1–1.5 cm wide.
Shape	Primary rhizome — ovate, oblong or pyriform. Secondary rhizome — more cylindrical.
Outer surface	Longitudinally wrinkled and transverse rings. Rings are also called scars or annulations.
Fractured surface	Waxy and resinous.
Fracture	Hard.

Organoleptic characters

Colour	Deep yellow to orange.
Odour	Slight.
Taste	Aromatic, pungent and bitter.

Chemical constituents

Colouring matters — curcuminoids, i.e. curcumin I (yellow), curcumin II and III. Volatile oils — zingeberine, phellandrine, borneol, cineole. Carbohydrates — glucose, fructose, starch, arabinose, etc.

Use

Aromatic, stomachic, carminative, blood purifier, stimulant and tonic.

Biological source

The given sample of crude drug consists of dried rhizome of *Curcuma longa* belonging to the family Zingiberaceae.

Experiment 33

OBJECT

Identification of root drug **Garlic** by morphological characters.

Synonyms

Lasan, allium.

Morphological characters

Type	Bulb, the bulb encloses several cloves in a silky white or pink membranous envelop.
Shape	The bulb is subglobular in shape where as cloves are flat and oval, joined with hard central axis.
Cloves	They are covered with scale leaves.

Organoleptic characters

Colour	Silky white.
Odour	Alliaceous.
Taste	Pungent and bitter.

Chemical constituents

The main constituent is allin. The other constituents are allicin, volatile oil, fatty oil, mucilage and albumin.

Use

Carminative, aphrodisiac, expectorant, stimulant. It is useful in treatment of cough bronchitis, asthma, whooping cough, tuberculosis and hypertension.

Biological source

The given sample of crude drug consists of dried bulb of *Allium sativum* belonging to the family Liliaceae.

Experiment 34

OBJECT

Identification of root drug **Rauwolfia** by morphological characters.

Synonyms

Sarpagandha, Indian snake root.

Morphological characters

Type	Rhizome and root.
Size, shape	8–15 cm long, 5–22 mm in diameter, cylindrical slightly tapering.
Outer surface	Greyish brown with faintly longitudinal ridges.
Fracture	Short, shows 3–8 growth rings.
Fractured surface	Yellow in colour.

Organoleptic characters

Odour	Odourless
Taste	Bitter

Chemical constituents

It contain alkaloids like reserpine, deserpidine, ajmalinine, ajamaline, ajmalicine, serpentine, etc. The other substances are phytosterols, fattyacid and sugars.

Use

Hypnotic, sedative, anti hypertensive agent, etc.

Biological source

The given sample of crude drug consists of dried roots and rhizome of *Rauwolfia serpentina* belonging to the family Apocynaceae.

Experiment 35

OBJECT

Identification of root drug **Rhubarb** by morphological characters.

Synonyms

Rheum, Revandchini.

Morphological characters

Type	Rhizome.
Size, Shape	5–15 cm in long, 3–8 cm in diameter, cylindrical or flat.
Surface	Outer–yellow in colour, smooth and showing white reticulations. Inner surface–shows many star spots and parallel radish orange lines.
Fracture	Irregular and granular.

Organoleptic characters

Taste	Astringent and bitter.

Chemical constituents

Anthraquinones glycosides: Chrysophenol, emodin, physcion, rhein, etc. The other constituents are glucogallin, catechin, calcium oxalate, etc.

Use

As laxative, stomachic, etc.

Biological source

The given sample of crude drug consists of dried roots and rhizomes of *Rheum officinale* belonging to the family Polygonaceae.

Experiment 36

OBJECT

Identification of root drug **Liquorice** by morphological characters.

Synonyms

Mulethi, Glycyrrhiza.

Morphological characters

Type	Peeled or unpeeled stolon and root.
Size, shape	5–30 cm in long, 1–2 cm in diameter. Peeled pieces — angular, Unpeeled pieces — straight, unbranched, cylindrical.
Surface	Outer — dark radish brown, longitudinally wrinkled Inner surface — straight, unbranched, cylindrical.
Fracture	Fibrous.
Wood	Splintery.
Stolons	Bears buds, scaly leaves and scars of lateral roots.

Organoleptic characters

Colour	Peeled–yellow, unpeeled–radish brown.
Odour	Faint and typical.
Taste	Sweet.

Chemical constituents

Glycyrrhizin, glycyrrhizihic acid, flavonoids, coumarins, betasitosterol, starch, protein, resin, glycycoumarine.

Use

Laxative, demulcent, diuretic, emmenagogue, etc. It is also used in treatment of cough, sore throat, genitourinary diseases, peptic ulcer, etc.

Biological source

The given sample of crude drug consists of dried unpeeled root and rhizome of *Glycyrrhiza glabra* belonging to the family Leguminosae.

Experiment 37

OBJECT

Identification of root drug **Picrorrhiza** by morphological characters.

Synonym

Kathi, Kuru.

Morphological characters

Size, Shape	2–4 cm long, 0.3–1 cm in diameter, sub-cylindrical and straight or slightly curved.
Surface	Longitudinally wrinkled, a few small root scars, numerous scale leaves.
Fracture	Short.
Fractured surface	Cork, xylem bundles, pith.

Organoleptic characters

Odour	Slightly unpleasant.
Taste	Very bitter.

Chemical constituents

Picrorhizin, kutkin, picrosides I, II and III, vanillic acid, mannitol, kutki sterol, apocyanin, etc.

Use

Bitter tonic, laxative, abortificient, etc. It is used in treatment of jaundice, kidney stone and skin disease.

Biological source

The given sample of crude drug consists of dried rhizome of *Picrorhiza kurroa* belonging to the family Scrophulariaceae.

Experiment 38

OBJECT

Identification of root drug **Shatavar** by morphological characters.

Synonym

Shatavari.

Morphological characters

Type	Fleshy tuberous.
Size, shape	5–15 cm long, 1–2 cm in diameter cylindrical and straight or slightly curved.
Surface	Wrinkled.
Fracture	Irregular.

Organoleptic characters

Colour	Wide to buff
Odour	Odourless
Taste	Bitter

Chemical constituents

Steroidal saponins—shatavarins I to IV. Aglycone unit is sarsapogenin.

Use

As refrigerant, demulcent, aphrodisiac, antiseptic, antidysenteric and galactagogue.

Biological source

The given sample of crude drug consists of dried root of *Asparagus racemosus* belonging to the family Liliaceae.

Experiment 39

OBJECT

Identification of root drug **Dioscorea** by morphological characters.

Synonyms

Wild yam, rheumatism root.

Morphological characters

Type	Tuber.
Stem	Slender, twening, glabrous.
Leaves	Alternate, foliolate, glabrous, petiolate, elliptic-lanceolate, acuminate, sub-caudate.
Male flower	Pale greenish, fragrant, racemes.
Bracts	Long and broad.
Perianth	Mottled with brown, ovate, subacute, sparsely, pubescent.
Stamens	3 perfect, pistilode – 3-lobed, capsules – quadrately oblong.
Seeds	Wing at the base.

Chemical constituents

Saponion glycoside diosgenin. It also contains small quantities of hecogenin and resin.

Use

Diosgenin is used for the production of various steroidal drugs like progesterone.

Biological source

The given sample of crude drug consists of dried root of *Dioscorea pentaphylla* and other species belonging to the family Dioscoreaceae.

Experiment 40

OBJECT

Identification of crude drug **Pippali** by morphological characters.

Synonym

Piplamul.

Morphological characters

Size	0.5–2.5 cm long, 2–7 mm in diameter.
Shape	Cylindrical, straight or slightly curved.
Root stock	Erect, thick, branched.
Stem	Numerous, ascending or prostrate, branched cylindrical and pubescent.
Leaves	Ovate, cordate, oblong, oval, cordate at base, sub acute, entire, reticulate venation, petiolate, stipulate, etc.
Spikes	Solitary, pedunculate.
Bracts	Narrow, stamens 2, stigma 3–4.
Perianth	Mottled with brown, ovate, subacute, sparsely pubescent.
Fruit	Very small, ovoid, completely sunk in solid fleshy spike which is 2.5–3.8 cm, ovoid-oblong, erect, blunt, blackish green, shiny, sweetish and pungent fruit.
Colour	Light brown.
Odour	Characteristics.
Taste	Bitter and pungent.

Chemical constituents

Alkaloids like piperine, piperlonguminine, piplartine, etc.

Use

As carminative sedative and tonic. It is also useful in treatment of cough, bronchitis, asthma and cold.

Biological source

The given sample of crude drug consists of cut pieces of root or underground stem or fruits of *Piper longum* and other species belonging to the family Piperaceae.

Experiment 41

OBJECT

Identification of root drug **Ipecacuanha** by morphological characters.

Synonym

Ipecac.

Morphological characters

Size, shape	5–15 cm long, 3–6 mm in diameter, cylindrical and tortous.
Surface	Annulated, ridges are rounded.
Fracture (root)	Short, shows thick greyish bark and small dense wood.
Fractured surface	The middle part is yellow in colour and edges are greyish in colour.

Organoleptic characters

Colour	Brown to brick red.
Odour	Slight.
Taste	Bitter and acrid.

Chemical constituents

Isoquinone alkaloids like emetine, cephaline, psychotrine. Besides these it also contains ipecacuanhin glycoside, starch, saponins, calcium oxalate, etc.

Use

As emetic, expectorant, diaphoretic, etc. It is useful in treatment of amoebic dysentery.

Biological source

The given sample of crude drug consists of dried root or rhizome of *Cephaelis ipecacuanha* belonging to the family Rubiaceae.

10

Herb and Whole Plant

Many plants and herbs as whole are got medicinal importance. Each part of the plant, i.e. stem, leaf, flower, fruit, etc. is used as drug, e.g. shankpuspi, punarnava, ephedra cannabis and vinea. Therefore morphology of herb and whole plant includes:

(a) The morphology of stem.
(b) The morphology of leaf.
(c) The morphology of flower.
(d) The morphology of fruit.

The morphology of each part, i.e. leaf, flower, fruit and stem has been discussed earlier in detail.

Experiment 42

OBJECT

Identification of herb drug **Shankhapushpi** by morphological characters.

Synonym

Vishnukranti.

Morphological characters (*Evolvulus alsinoides*)

Type	Perennial herb.
Size, shape (leaves)	2.5–3 cm long, filiform.
Stem	Woody and prostrate, about 30 cm long, hairy.
Leaves	Type — simple, petiole — sessile, arrangement — alternate, shape — lanceolate to suborbicular.
Flower	Small, blue in colour, solitary, long peduncles, axillary.
Fruit	Four-angled capsule.

Convolvulus pluricaulis

Condition	Shrub.
Stem	woody at the base.
leaves	shape — linear, oblong tapering at base, size — 2.5–3 cm long.
Flower	Small, funnel shaped, pink or white in colour.
Fruit	Small, glabrous, scarcely papillose.

Chemical constituents

Shankhapushpine alkaloid, volatile oil, triancontane, fatty alcohol, kaempferol, Betasitosterol, carbohydrate, protein, tannins, etc.

Use

As brain tonic, anthelmintic and febrifuse. It is also useful in treatment of hypertension, dysentery and bronchitis.

Biological source

The given sample of crude drug consists of the whole aerial parts of *Convolvulus pluricaulis* and *Evolvulus alsinoides* and other species belonging to the family Convolvulaceae.

Experiment 43

OBJECT

Identification of herb drug **Punarnava** by morphological characters.

Synonyms

Hogweed, Beshakapori.

Morphological characters

Type	Perennial herb.
Size, shape (leaves)	25–30 cm long, ovate-oblong.
Stem	Greenish purple in colour, cylindrical pubescent, prostrate, thickened at nodes
Leaves	Apex — rounded or slightly pointed. Base — subcordated or rounded. Arrangement — opposite. Lamina — glabrous and green above whitish below. Margin — entire.
Flower	Small, umbel inflorescence, bract and bractioles present. Perianth — in form of tube. Colour — pink.
Fruit	One-seeded.

Chemical constituents

Alkaloids like punarnavine, xanthine, etc. betasitosterol, fattyacid, potassium nitrate and potassium sulphate.

Use

As diuretic, clinically used in nephrotic syndrome, chronic oedema and liver diseases.

Biological source

The given sample of crude drug consists of the herb of *Boerhaavia diffusa* belonging to the family Nyctaginaceae.

Experiment 44

OBJECT

Identification of herb drug **Ephedra** by morphological characters.

Synonym

Ma-haung.

Morphological characters

Stem	Erect, woody, nodes and inter nodes present, cylindrical, brown in colour.
Leaves	Arrangement — opposite. Apex— subulate and recurved. Lamina — whitish.
Base of lamina	Reddish brown.

Organoleptic characters

Odour	Odourless
Taste	Bitter

Chemical constituents

The chief alkaloid is ephedrine. The other alkaloids are pseudoephedrine, 1-methyl ephedrine, nor-ephedrine, etc.

Use

Asthma, hay fever, rhinitis. The decoction is used for rheumatism and syphilis. Tincture is useful as cardiac and circulatory stimulant.

Biological source

The given sample of crude drug consists of whole aerial parts of *Ephedra sinica* and other species, belonging to the family Ephedraceae.

Experiment 45

OBJECT

Identification of crude drug **Cannabis** by morphological characters.

Synonyms

Ganja, charas, Indian hemp, bhang.

Morphological characters

Condition	Flattened rough, green masses. Dried resin is hard, brittle and does not stick.
Stem	Erect, slender, cylindrical longitudinally furrowed, pale brown to pale green in colour.
Leaves	Stalked, palmate, alternate.
Bract	Numerous, up to 1.5 cm long, alternate, stipulate.
Bracteoles	Boat shaped with acute pieces, incurved at the base to enclose the flower or fruit.
Flower	Yellow in colour, ovary enclosed by a hairy perianth.
Ovary	2 mm long, thread like, two thin styles brownish red colour.
Fruit	5–6 mm long, 4 mm wide, type — achenes, ovoid, glossy green or yellowish green in colour, enclosed in the persistent perianth with single seed.

Chemical constituents

Semi solid resin. It contains various cannabinoids like cannabinol, cannabidiol, cannabidiol — carboxylic acid, cannabigerol and tatrahydrocannabinols (Δ^8, Δ^9-THC) which possesses euphoric activity. The other constituents are volatile oil, choline, calcium carbonate and trigonelline.

Use

As narcotic, anticonvulsant, anti-anxiety, antispasmodic. It causes euphoria, delusion, hallucinations and drowsiness.

Biological source

The given sample of crude drug consists of dried flowering tops of pistillate plants of *Cannabis sativa* belonging to the family Moraceae.

Experiment 46

OBJECT

Identification of crude drug **Vinca** by morphological characters.

Synonyms

Shadaphul, Rattanjot.

Morphological characters

Condition	Herb or sub-shrub.
Stem	Woody at base.
Leaves	Oblong, petiolate. Base — acute. Apex — rounded. Margin — entire.
Flower	Axillary, violate, pink or white flower, 4–5 cm in diameter.
Fruit	Divergent follicle.
Odour	Slight.
Taste	Bitter.

Chemical constituents

Indole alkaloids — vincristine, vinblastine, catharanthine, ajmalicine, reserpine, serpentine. Besides these it also contains monoterpines sesquiterpenes, indole glycosides.

Use

Leukaemia, Hodgkin's disease diabetes, and wasp sting.

Biological source

The given sample of crude drug consists of whole plant or aerial parts of *Catharanthus roseus* (*Vinca rosea*) belonging to the family Apocynaceae.

11

Wood

Woods consists of xylem and the mainly secondary xylem formed by the activity of the cambium.

There are two types of cambium.

1. *Fascicular (intrafascicular) cambium:* It is primary meristem which is found between phloem and primary xylem.
2. *Interfescicular cambium:* It is secondary meristem which develops outside the vascular bundle. The cambium activity varies greatly by the changes of climate. The band of xylem produced in autumn or summer is called autumn wood or summer wood respectively. The cambium grows much actively in spring session and produces spring wood.

Heart wood and sap wood

In woody stem, the older part of the xylem becomes non functional because they get filled with resin, gummy or tannin like substances and tyloses. These are formed as a result of compression of thin-walled living cells during enormous secondary growth.

So the central portion of non functional xylem is called heart wood which is dark in colour and stores various kinds of products. The outer young and functional parts of xylem is called sap wood. The conversion of sap wood in to heart wood is a progressive phenomenon which continue throughout the life of the plant.

S. No.	*Heart wood (duramen)*	*Sap wood (alburnum)*
1.	It is central dark coloured nonfunctional part of secondary xylem.	It is outer light coloured functional part of secondary xylem.
2.	Parenchymatous cells of heartwood are dead.	Parenchymatous cells of sap wood are living.
3.	Tyloses, resin, gum or tannin are present.	These are absent.
4.	It is more heavier and durable.	It is lighter and less durable.
5.	It is less susceptible to the attack of pathogens and insects.	It is more susceptible to the attack of pathogens and insects

S. No.	*Spring wood (early wood)*	*Autumn wood (late wood)*
1.	Formation of xylem in favourable condition.	Formation of xylem in unfavourable condition.
2.	Quantity of xylem is more.	Quantity of xylem is less.
3.	The tracheary elements of xylem are thin-walled with wide lumen.	The tracheary elements of xylem are thick-walled with narrow lumen.

The morphology of woods

It includes the following description.

1. Colour and density
2. Annual rings
3. Vessels
4. Medullary rays
5. Wood parenchyma
6. Odour and taste

Experiment 47

OBJECT

Identification of wood drug **Sandal wood** by morphological characters.

Synonym

Chandan wood.

Type

Heart wood.

Colour and density

Yellowish and pale reddish, hard, heavy and dense.

Annual rings

Alternating lighter and darker zones.

Medullary rays

Very fine and close together.

Vessels

Mostly solitary being only occasionally arranged in small radial groups.

Taste

Slightly bitter.

Odour

Strong and fragrant.

Chemical constituents

santalol, santene, santalenes, santenol, santalone.

Use

In perfumery and stimulant.

The given sample of crude drug consists of heart wood of *Santalum album* belonging to family Santalaceae.

12

Gross Anatomical Study

Gross anatomical studies (TS) of the following drugs:

1. *Leaves:* Senna, datura.
2. *Bark:* Cinnamon, cinchona.
3. *Fruit:* Coriander, fennel.
4. *Flower:* Clove.
5. *Seed:* Nux vomica.
6. *Rhizome:* Ginger, ipecacuanha.

The tissue system

There are mainly three tissue systems in plant.

1. Epidermal system.
2. Ground tissue system.
3. Vascular (fascicular) system.

Epidermal system

It originates from apical meristem.

(a) Epidermis

The epidermal cells are generally compactly arranged. The cells are parenchymatous and living.

(b) Cuticle

A fatty substance cutin is deposited over the outer surface of epidermal cells. The cuticle layer may be thin or thick and smooth or rough.

(c) Stomata

They consist of two kidney-shaped guard cells surrounding a pore. In some species guard cells are surrounded by subsidiary cells. The guard cells usually have thick walled towards pore and thin walled on opposite side.

(d) Trichomes

These are epidermal out growth. They may be unicellular or multicellular.

Functions of epidermal tissue system

1. It forms covering of all the plant parts and therefore provides protection.
2. It helps in reduction of surface evaporation of water due to presence of cuticle.
3. The epidermis forms phellogen by introduction of meristematic activity. It gives rise to cork layers and also helps in healing of wounds.
4. All gaseous exchange occurs through stomata and lenticels present in the epidermis.

Ground tissue system

It forms the bulk of body and consists of mainly parenchymatous, collenchymatous, sclerenchymatous, glandular and laticeferous tissue. This tissue system originates from ground meristem.

1. Cortex

It is the region between the epidermis and endodermis. This region consists of primary cells, specially parenchymatous, collenchymatous and sclerenchymatous. The main functions of cortex are storage of water, reserve food, to provide turgidity to the plant body, lateral transport of minerals, organic solutes and water, to provide mechanical support and gaseous exchange.

2. Endodermis

It is a single layer of compactly arranged parenchymatous cells present between the cortex and pericycle.

3. Pericycle

It is single layered or multi layered cylinder of thin-walled or thick-walled cells present between the epidermis and vascular tissues. In dicot. roots the cork cambium originates in the pericycle which results in the formation periderm.

4. Medullary rays

The primary medullary rays are present in between the adjacent vascular bundle in primary structure of dicot. stem. These are made up of parenchymatous cells and extend from pith towards the periphery.

5. Pith

It is centrally located tissues, is made up of parenchymatous cells with intracellular spaces. It stores water and food.

6. Ground tissue of leaves

Ground tissue of petiole is made up of uniform parenchymatous cells with distinct intercellular spaces, in leaf lamina the bulk of ground tissue is called mesophyll which is usually differentiated into palisade and spongy parenchyma. The main function of mesophyll is photosynthesis.

Vascular tissue system

This tissue system includes vascular tissues, i.e. xylem and phloem. The xylem and phloem strands are usually found in bundles called vascular bundles.

Radial

The xylem and phloem are found in different radious, e.g. roots.

Conjoint

A vascular bundle having both xylem and phloem together is called conjoint, e.g. stem.

Collateral

A vascular bundle in which the phloem lies towards outside and xylem toward inner side.

Bicollateral

A vascular bundle having the phloem strands are both outer and inner side of xylem.

Concentric

One tissue is completely surrounded by the other.

(a) Amphivasal: The phloem lies in the centre and is surrounded by xylem.

(b) Amphicribal: The xylem lies in the centre and is surrounded by phloem.

Open vascular bundle

The cambium is present.

Closed vascular bundle

The cambium is absent.

Exarch

The protoxylem lies towards periphery and metaxylem towards centre.

Endarch

The protoxylem lies towards centre and metaxylem towards periphery.

Mesarch

The protoxylem remains surrounded on all sides by metaxylem.

Section cutting

The nature and arrangement of tissue system can be studied conveniently by cutting thin sections of plant parts transversely and longitudinally. Hold the material being examined between the first finger and thumb of the left hand. The position of the thumb should be just below the surface of the material to avoid injury to the finger. Take the razor in the right hand and cut the number of sections. Put all sections in watch glass containing water. The section cutting of the lamina of the leaf is carried out by sandwiching the material between the two pieces of pith or potato. Take a clean slide and place a drop of glycerine water in the centre of the slide. Select the thin section of material and put it on the slide. Place cover slip on the material being examined without any air bubbles trapped inside. Focus the slides containing material under the microscope and adjust the require illumination with the help of condenser and diaphragm.

Experiment 48

OBJECT

To study the histology of **Senna** leaf by transverse section cutting.

Histology

1. Epidermis

It is made up of polygonal cells with straight anticlinal walls. The epidermis cells contain mucilage. The cells of lower epidermis are smaller with thick cuticle.

2. Stomata

Paracytic type of stomata on both surfaces.

3. Epidermal trichomes

Unicellular, conical thick walled with warty cuticle.

4. Mesophyll

(i) **Upper palisade:** Compact, elongated cells in single layer.
(ii) **Spongy mesophyll:** Loosely arranged parenchymatous cells between upper and lower palisade.
(iii) **Lower palisade:** Cells are smaller than that of upper palisade. There are loosely arranged with wavy walls.

5. Meristele

A radiate xylem and phloem with and arc of pericyclic fibres.

6. Calcium oxalate

Crystals are found in palisade and spongy tissue.

7. Midrib

Biconvex, collenchymatous cells.

8. Vascular bundle

Collateral vascular bundle and covered by sclerenchymatous fibres.

Experiment 49

Object

To study the histology of **Datura** leaf by transverse section cutting.

Histology

1. Epidermis

- (i) **Cuticle:** On both surfaces.
- (ii) **Epidermal trichomes:** *Datura innoxia* has glandular trichomes where as the leaf of *Datura metel* have covering trichomes.
- (iii) **Stomata:** The numbers of both surface are nearly equal. Anesocytic type of stomata is found.
- (iv) **Upper epidermis:** The rectangular cells are arranged in single layer.
- (v) **Lower epidermis:** Wavy walled cells.

2. Mesophyll

- (i) **Palisade:** Elongated cells, single layer and compact.
- (ii) **Spongy parenchyma:** Loosely arranged multilayered. It contains sphaeraphides and microsphenoidal crystals also.

3. Midrib

Bicollateral vascular bundle, collenchymatous layer is followed by parenchyma cells containing microsphenoidal crystals and calcium oxalate.

Experiment 50

OBJECT

To study the histology of **Cinchona** bark by transverse section cutting.

Histology

1. Periderm

(i) **Cork:** Multilayered thin-walled cells, impregnated with suberin.
(ii) **Cork Cambium (phellogen):** 2–3 layers followed by 6–8 layers of phelloderm.
(iii) **Phelloderm:** 6–8 layers forming the cortex.

2. Cortex

Multilayered thin walled parenchymatous cells containing starch grains and microcrystals of calcium oxalate.

3. Secondary Phloem

(i) **Pholem fibres:** Spindle-shaped thick lignified wall containing funnel shaped pits, fusiform, yellow in colour.
(ii) **Phloem parenchyma**
(iii) **Sieve tubes with companion cells**
(iv) **Medullary rays:** 1–3 seriate, radially elongated thin walled cells.

Experiment 51

OBJECT

To study the histology of **Cinnamon** bark by transverse section cutting.

Histology

1. Pericyclic fibres 6–15 in groups, lignified sclerenchymatous.
2. Sclereids horse shoe shaped thickened lignified wall containing starch grains.
3. Phloem fibres single or groups of 3–4, lignified.
4. Meullary rays uni or biseriate, radially elongated possessing crystals of calcium oxalate.
5. Sieve tubes—tangentially arranged.
6. Phloem parenchyma—sub-rectangular, thin walled cells containing starch grains and calcium oxalate.
7. Secretary cells—elongated containing volatile oil and mucilage.

Experiment 52

OBJECT

To study the histology of **Coriander** fruit by transverse section cutting.

Histology

1. Epicarp	Polygonal tabular cells with occasional stomata, a single prism of calcium oxalate is reported in each cell.
2. Mesocarp	An outer and an inner layer of parenchyma with fusiform and lignified sclerenchymatous cells in between. The rows (outer and inner) are arranged longitudinally and tangentially.
3. Vittae	Two on commissural surface and four on dorsal surface.
4. Endocarp	Characteristic appearance of parquetry cells.
5. Endosperm	Cellulosic parenchyma shows presence of oil globules and aleurone grains.
6. Trichomes	Absent.

Experiment 53

OBJECT

To study the histology of **Fennel** by transverse section cutting.

Histology

1. Epicarp	Polygonal cells with smooth cuticle.
2. Mesocarp	**(i) V. Bundle** 5 in number, bicollateral, reticulate and lignified parenchyma surrounded by the vascular bundles. **(ii) Vittae** 4 on the dorsal surface and two on the commissural surface.
3. Endocarp	Parquetry arranged cells in a single layer between mesocarp and testa.
4. Testa	Yellow in single layer.
5. Endosperm	Thick-walled parenchyma with oil globules and aleurone grains.
6. Embryo	Crescent-shaped.
7. Raphae	In the middle of commissural surface in front of carpophore.

Experiment 54

OBJECT

To study the histology of flower bud of **Clove** by transverse section cutting.

Histology

A TS through hypanthium

1. Epidermis — Single layer with thick cuticle (anomocytic) ranunculaceous type of stomata.

2. Cotex

(a) Peripheral region

- **(i) Parenchyma:** Radially elongated containing ellipsoidal schizolysigenous oil glands.
- **(ii) VB:** Bicollateral, about 15 in number.
- **(iii) Calcium oxalate crystals:** Present in cluster.

(b) Middle region

- **(i) Pericyclic fibres.**
- **(ii) Xylem:** 3–5 lignified spiral vessels.
- **(iii) Aerenchyma:** A zone of aerenchyma within the ring of vascular bundles.

(c) Central region (Columella)

Thick walled parenchymatous cells with cluster crystal of calcium oxalate, vascular bundles (20–25) and numerous sphaeraphides.

A TS through region of ovary

Dessepiment of ovary — Parenchymatous
Placentation — axile

Experiment 55

OBJECT

To study the histology of rhizome **Ginger** by transverse section cutting.

Histology

1. Cork

- **(a) Outer zone:** Irregular arranged parenchymatous cells.
- **(b) Inner zone:** Radially arranged parenchymatous cells.

2. Cotex

Thick walled rounded parenchymatous cells with intercellular spaces.

- **(a) Starch grains:** Ovoid or sack-shaped in cortex.
- **(b) Oil glands and oleoresin:** Yellowish brown oleoresin and numerous oil glands are found in the cortex.

3. Endodermis

A single layer.

4. Ground tissue

Parenchymatous polygonal cells with abundant starch, oleo-resin and v. bundles.

5. Pericycle

A single layer.

6. VB

Collateral, conjoint, nonlignified fibres.

7. Xylem vessels

Annular, spiral or reticulate.

Experiment 56

OBJECT

To study the histology of **Nux vomica** seed by transverse section cutting.

Histology

1. Epidermis

Hairy, thick-walled lignified cells.

2. Trichomes

Thick-walled lignified slightly bent. The inner region of testa consists of collapsed cells.

3. Endodermis

Thick-walled cellulosic, parenchyma, iso-diametric cells. It contains aleurone grains and fixed oil globules.

4. Endosperm

(a) **Outer part:** Brucin.
(b) **Inner part:** Strychnine.

5. Plasmodesma

Very fine protoplasmic threads of the endosperm cells which communicate through the cell walls.

Experiment 57

OBJECT

To study the histology of **Ipecacuanha** root by transverse section cutting.

Histology

1. Periderm

- **(a) Cork:** Thin, brown, tangentially elongated cells.
- **(b) Phellogen:** In two layers below the cork.
- **(c) Phelloderm:** Wide rounded cells (cellulosic parenchyma containing starch and calcium oxalate).

2. Phloem

Parenchymatous cells with perforated sieve tubes and no fibres.

3. Xylem

Secondary xylem contain vessels and tracheids with bordered pits. Xylem parenchyma has simple pits and starch.

4. Medullary rays

Radially elongated containing starch grain.

13

Identification of Fibres and Surgical Dressing

Fibres (natural and artificial) are used in surgical dressings.

Classification of fibres

1. Vegetable fibres, e.g. cotton, jute.
2. Animal fibres, e.g. wool, silk.
3. Mineral fibres, e.g. glass, asbestos.
4. Synthetic fibres, e.g. nylon.
5. Regenerated fibres.
   (a) Carbohydrate, e.g. rayon.
   (b) Protein: Fibrolin.

IDENTIFICATION OF FIBRES

It can be carried out by chemical test and microscopical examination.

Microscopic characters

Vegetable fibres and regenerated fibres

Absorbent cotton: Unicellular, flattened and twisted with round apex.
Jute (Phloem fibres): Yellowish brown, bluntly pointed or rounded.
Regenerated carbohydrate: Transparent with slight twist grooves along their length.

Wool

Presence of cuticle and medulla, elongated fusiform cells of cortex.

Silk

Lack of cellular structures.

Experiment 58

OBJECT

To identify the different types of fibres by physical, chemical test and report.

Vegetable and regenerated fibres

Physical and chemical tests

S. No.	*Test*	*Procedure*
1.	Solubility	Ab. cotton is insoluble in warm HCl, 60% warm KOH and 5% H_2SO_4, phenol, etc. Rayon and Jute–It is soluble in 60% H_2SO_4
2.	Ignition	Burn without odour.
3.	N/50 Iodine and 80% H_2SO_4	Rayon and absorbent cottons take blue stain.
4.	Molish's test (Solution of naphthol in H_2SO_4)	They give violet colour.
5.	Chlorzinc iodine or solution of iodine and sulphuric acid	Absorbent cottons and rayon produce blue stain whereas jute gives yellow stain.
6.	Cuoxam (copper oxide ammonia solution)	Absorbent cottons — swell, dissolve Jute — insoluble Rayon — swells, dissolves
7.	Million's reagent and picric acid	They give negative test.

Physical and chemical tests of animal fibres and synthetic

S. No.	*Test*		*Procedure*	
1.	Solubility	5% KOH, Warm	Wool–Soluble	Silk–Sparingly soluble
		Warm HCl	Wool–Insoluble Nylon–Soluble	Silk–Soluble
		60% H_2SO_4	Wool–Insoluble Nylon–Slightly Soluble	Silk–Soluble
		Formic acid, phenol 90%, HNO_3 70%	Nylon–Soluble	
2.	Ignition	Animal fibres	Burns slowly with foul odour	
		Synthetic	Hard bead formation	
3.	N/50 Iodine and 80% H_2SO_4.	Wool, silk	Yellowish brown	
		Synthetic	Negative	
4.	Picric acid	Wool	Deep yellow	
		Silk	Yellow	
5.	Million's reagent	Wool, silk	Brick red	
6.	Lead acetate alkaline, boil	Wool	Blackens	
		Synthetic	Negative	
7.	Cuoxam test	Wool	Blue, insoluble	
		Silk	soluble	
		Synthetic	Negative	

Result

14

Physical and Chemical Tests for Evaluation of Unorganized Drugs

Drugs, which are uniform, and a cellular products are called *unorganized drugs*. These drugs are obtained from parts of plants or animals by some processes of extractions like.

1. Incision – e.g. opium
2. Decoction – e.g. agar
3. Expression – e.g. olive oil
4. Natural secretions – e.g. bees wax, myrrh

Broadly these drugs can be divided into the following two categories:

1. Solids – e.g. gums, resins, etc.
2. Liquids – e.g. balsams and oils (fixed and essential)

These drugs cannot be classified morphologically but can be classified on the basis of method of their origin and nature as follows.

A. Plant products

1. Dried latex – e.g. opium
2. Dried juice – e.g. aloes
3. Extracts – e.g. catechu, agar
4. Gums – e.g. acacia, tragacanth
5. Resins – e.g. colophony, asafetida, benzoin, guggal
6. Oleo–gum–resins – e.g. myrrh, copaiba.
7. Waxes – e.g. bees wax
8. Saccharine substances – e.g. honey
9. Fats and oils (fixed and essential) e.g. castor oil, oil of clove, essential oil, etc.

B. Animal products

1. Fats and oils – e.g. cod liver oil, shark liver oil
2. Proteins – e.g. gelatin

Latex

These are the emulsions of suspensions in which continuous phase is aqueous solution of mineral salts, sugar or proteins, etc. and suspended particles are oil drops resins, gums, etc. The turbid fluid is normally white in colour.

Extract

These are prepared by evaporation of aqueous decoctions of certain parts of plants/animal.

Juices

Drugs in liquid form obtained by compression of certain parts of plants, e.g. dried juice obtained from cut leaves of aloe and dried latex obtained from capsule of poppy.

Gums

These are exudates obtained by producing incisions in bark, these are amorphous, translucent solid substance, these are soluble in water and produce viscous, adhesive solution with water or swollen in water to form jelly like mass. These are in soluble in alcohol and many organic solvents. These are abnormal pathological products of plants produced due to pathological condition brought about by injury, etc.

Resins

These are heterogeneous mixture of chemical substances, which include acids, esters, glycosides and resenes. These are heavier than water, usually amorphous, hard and a brittle solid, on heating softens and fuse, insoluble in water, more or less soluble in alcohol, organic solvents and fixed and volatile oil, these are classified as

- Acid resins – e.g. colophony, guaiacum
- Ester resins – e.g. benzoin
- Mixed resins – e.g. shellac

Oleo–gum–resins: As the name indicate the substances chiefly consists of resins with gum (gum–resins), e.g. myrrh or resins with volatile oils or oily liquid (olio- resins), e.g. balsams.

Waxes

Normally solid, physically similar to fats and oils, but chemically differ, consisting of mixture of esters or of esters and acids, but never contains ester of glycerol.

Fixed oils and fats

These are substances obtained from vegetable or animals, liquids are known as oils and solids are known as "fat", lighter than water, greasy, insoluble in water. Freely soluble in ether, chloroform but usually soluble in alcohol, do not volatile in air, chemically these are esters of glycerol which is combined with organic acid of high molecular weight.

Saccharine substances

These substances are normally solid or liquid, translucent, and soluble in water. Sweet in taste either a result of exudation of plant (e.g. Manna) or made by animal (e.g. honey).

Experiment 59

OBJECT

Identification of unorganized drug **Aloes** by study of physical and chemical characters.

Synonyms

Ghee, Gwar, Gwarpatha.

Physical characters

Physical form	Solid, waxy mass.
Colour and fluorescence	Dark brown opaque.
Hardness and fracture	Hard, uneven porous fracture.
Viscosity	Before drying juice is very viscous.
Solubility	Soluble in alcohol and miscible with water.
Effect of heat	At high temperature produce black mass.
Odour and Taste	Characteristic unpleasant odour, very bitter and nauseous taste.

Chemical tests

Boil 0.5 g with 50 ml water until nearly dissolved, cool and add 0.5 g kieselguhr and filter, apply the following tests to the filtrate.

1. Borax test

Heat 5 ml of filtrate with 0.2 g of borax until dissolved, then add few drops of this solution to a test tube nearly filled with water : Green fluorescence is produced due to hydrolysis of barbaloin which liberate aloe-emodin anthranol.

2. Bromine test

A pale yellow copious precipitate of tetrabromoaloin is obtained when above filtrate mixed with freshly prepared bromine solution equally.

3. Nitric Acid test

A yellowish brown colour to a vivid green is produced with cape aloes and a deep brownish-red colour with curacao aloes (socotrine–pale brown yellow; Zanzibar–pale yellowish-brown) when 5 ml of filtrate mixed with 2 ml of nitric acid.

4. Cupraloin test for isobarbaloin

To 10 ml of 0.1% solution of aloes in distilled water, add 1 drop of 5% solution of copper acetate, 0.5 ml of saturated solution of sodium chloride, 1 ml of alcohol and warm : Deep wine red colour with curacao aloes, pale wine red colour with cape aloes. Socotrine and Zanzibar do not give colour.

Use

Used as purgative and improve digestion.

Biological source

The given sample of crude drug consists of dried juice of various sp. of *Aloes* family Liliaceae.

Experiment 60

OBJECT

Identification of unorganized drug **Catechu** by physical and chemical characters.

Synonym

Kattha.

Physical characters

Physical form	Solid mass.
Colour and fluorescence	Externally dull dark reddish brown, internally pale yellow.
Hardness and fracture	Hard, friable, break easily in porous fractures.
Solubility	Slightly soluble in alcohol and water.
Odour and taste	Odourless, very bitter astringent after sweetish taste.

Chemical tests

1. Catechu tannic acid present produces green, blue or black colour with solution of ferric chloride.
2. Prepare alcoholic solution of catechu, make it alkaline with caustic soda, shake with light petroleum, a brilliant green fluorescence is produced.
3. Dip the match stick in decoction of catechu, dry it and again dip in conc. HCl . Dry again and burn in flame. It gives pink or red or violet coloured flame due to formation of phloroglucinol.
4. Prepare the vanillin–HCl–Alcohol reagent in ratio of 1:10:10. Catechu gives pink or red colour with above reagent in warm condition.

The black catechu gives all the test except test number 2 (fluorescence test) which distinguishes it from pale catechu.

Use

used as astringent in diarrhoea and as local astringent in lozenges.

Biological source

The given sample of crude drug (pale catechu) consists of dried extract from leaves of *Uncaria gambier* family Rubiaceae. Where as black catechu is dried extract from the heart wood of *Acacia catechu* family Leguminosae.